LIFE SUCKS:

How To Make It Better?

by **The Warrior**

Copyright © 2020 by The Warrior

All rights reserved. This book or any portion thereof may not be reproduced or used in any manner whatsoever without the express written permission of the publisher except for the use of brief quotations in a book review.

For anyone who's fighting a difficult battle in life.

CONTENTS

INTRODUCTION	- 7 -
THE MEANING OF CHALLENGES	- 11 -
HOW TO ACCEPT THINGS THE WAY THEY ARE	- 22 -
THE MOST IMPORTANT LOVE	- 31 -
DETACHING FROM NEGATIVE FEELINGS	- 46 -
THE CURE OF DESIRES	- 55 -
FINDING ONE'S LIFE PURPOSE	- 71 -
WALKING TO ULTIMATE HAPPINESS	- 82 -
TAKING CONTROL IN THE FACE OF ADVERSITY	- 92 -
THE ANTIDOTE OF HATE	- 100 -
OVERCOMING LAZINESS AND PROCRASTINATION	- 108 -
THE ONLY PATH TO SUCCESS	- 115 -
FINAL WORDS	- 128 -
RECOMMENDED READING	- 132 -

INTRODUCTION

Are you going through a difficult time in life?

Are you overwhelmed by inner turmoil and negative emotions?

Are you looking for your happiness and purpose of living?

Or struggling with laziness and procrastination that stop you from achieving your dreams?

If yes, then it's important that you can take a step back and discover yourself. It's important that you can deal with the inner turmoil before you can devise a plan and create a happier future.

"Life Sucks: How to make it better" will help you:

- Enhance your self-worth and confidence.

- Deal with your fears, stress, anxiety and depression.

- Overcome difficult times in life.

- Find out your life purpose.

- Create lasting happiness and fulfillment.

- Take control of your own life.

- Defeat laziness and procrastination.

- Work your way to ultimate success.

- Become the person you want to be.

- And much more.

Truth is, we cannot change what already happened to us. We cannot change how excruciating and devastating our painful past came to be. But we can always take control of our thoughts and actions, from this moment onwards. We can always create new plans and work our way towards a better future.

We Can Make It!

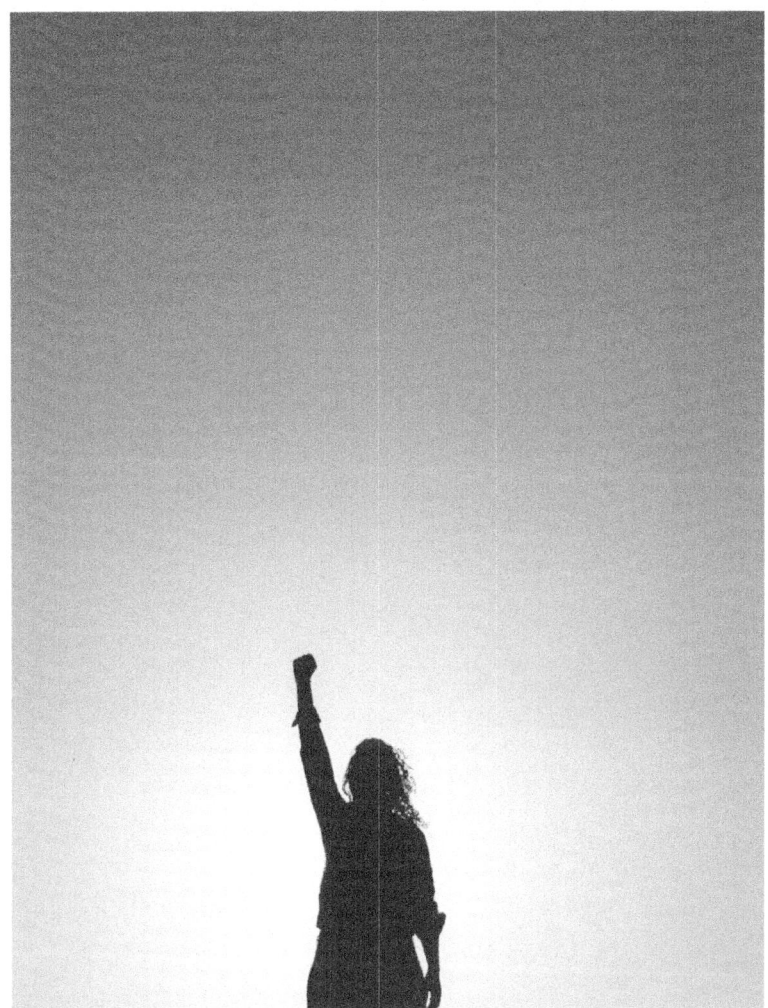

1

THE MEANING OF CHALLENGES

The pessimist sees difficulty in every opportunity. The optimist sees the opportunity in every difficulty.

- **Winston Churchill**

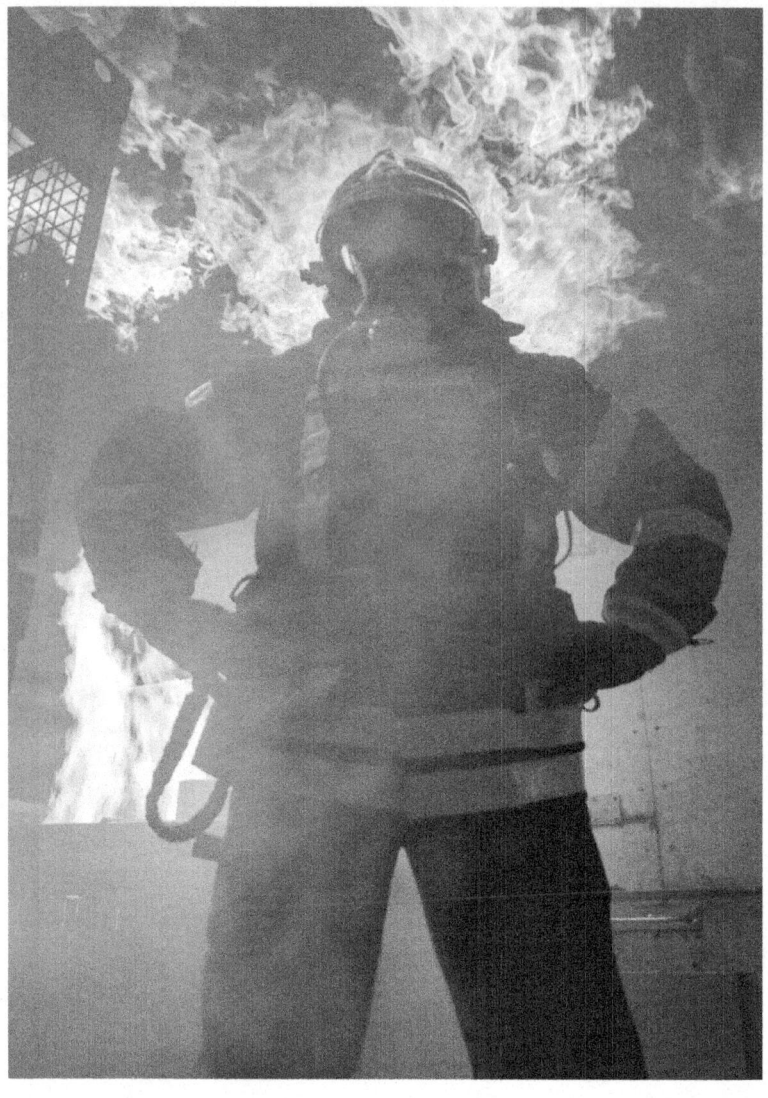

Our lives always have many ups and downs.

As often, after overcoming one problem in life, we shortly encounter another. Without stepping back and have a broader perspective, then, it's very easy to fall into the vicious cycle of stress and negativity. "Gosh, how could I get out of this?" We constantly trouble our minds with those nagging problems, feeling powerless against the world and its misfortunes.

Normally, we define a problem as something that goes against our expectations. When everything happens as expected, we feel satisfied. However, when a situation doesn't happen the way we wish, we feel negative about life and struggle against it.

Often, problems occur when we don't expect them. As that happens, we have only two options. Either we keep complaining, blaming the situation and doing nothing. Or, we can take the challenge as an opportunity, do something to tackle it and improve our life.

Although problems often bring us discomfort, or even extreme pains and miseries in life, we need to have them to master ourselves and grow up. We sometimes need to harden ourselves before life has the opportunity to destroy us.

The question is, why are challenges necessary for a happy life?

Because challenges could inspire us.

Hardships and difficulties often force people to look at themselves and the world from a newer perspective. They also force people to go out of their comfort zone and find out a better solution. Challenges therefore are meant to help us expand ourselves and learn necessary life skills. Indeed, the ability to overcome hardships and invent new tools is what has made our human species the conqueror and the master of this world.

Challenges help us find out who we are

Life is like a journey in which we strive to find out who we are and discover our fullest potentials. Challenges and hardships are in fact opportunities that help us realize how strong and resilient we can be. They let us grow and achieve our highest potentials that we could never think of. It's often said that if something can't kill you, it will make you stronger. Only when we stop running away from problems and confront them head-on can we get stronger and fully enjoy each day in life.

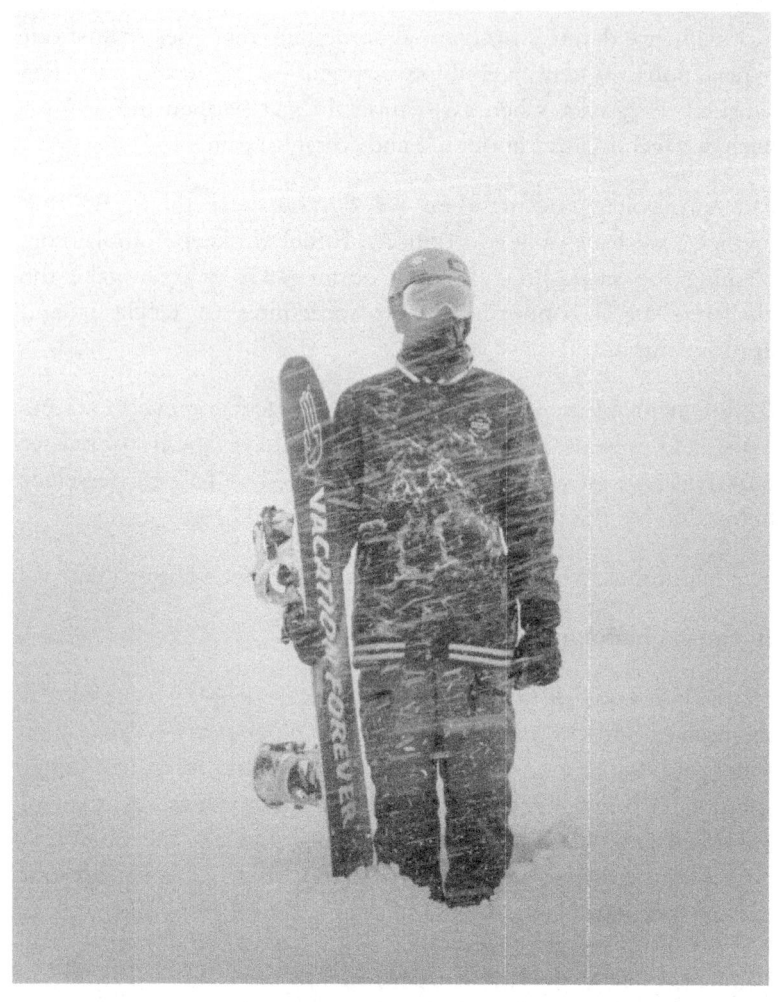

Overcoming challenges helps us discover our purpose

Hardships and challenges force us to step back, have a broader perspective, and help us realize what truly matters and what doesn't. They help us become aware of our ultimate purpose to strive for in life. That way, we'll have a clearer direction and motivation to move relentlessly forward, and know exactly how to enrich our lives with burning excitement and powerful meaning.

And conquering challenges gives us more confidence

Confidence is intimately related to people's experiences. Specifically, it's related to how much people believe they can overcome difficulties and achieve their goals. It's related to how much they believe in their capabilities and potentials. Truth is, to discover one's power and achieve confidence in life, a person has to face challenges and overcome them. Problems and hardships are therefore necessary ingredients for a greater life. They are necessary ingredients for a greater sense of one's worth.

Consider the inspiring story of W Mitchell.

On July 19, 1971, Mitchell encountered a tragic motorcycle accident in San Francisco. His face and body were brutally burned. His fingers were severely deformed that he lost almost all of them.

Not defeated by this painful accident, Mitchell fought bravely with the new challenges. He accepted and adapted to his new body. At last, he could recover from the accident and return to his normal life.

On November 11, 1975, unfortunately, Mitchell was involved in a disastrous plane crash. His spinal cord was severely injured, leaving him paralyzed from the waist down. He was sentenced to life in a wheelchair afterwards.

Surrendered and got destroyed by his tragic fate? Not at all!

Mitchell moved forward with his life step by step. He focused constantly on what he could still control, and ignored all the uncontrollable. Mitchell became a great businessman who created works for many people, a congressional nominee and an active environmentalist. He has been a host for many television shows, a well-known author, and an inspiring international speaker.

Today, Mitchell empowers and inspires millions of people with his story. He motivates others to confront challenges, embrace uncertainty and take well-planned action. Mitchell proves that unexpected challenges can turn into a powerful new starting point. He is one of the most inspiring people in the world, a heroic example of fighting without surrendering.

"Before I was paralyzed there were 10,000 things I could do. Now there are 9,000. I can either dwell on the 1,000 I've lost or focus on the 9,000 I have left." – **W Mitchell**

Talk about a powerful perspective to embrace challenges in one's life!

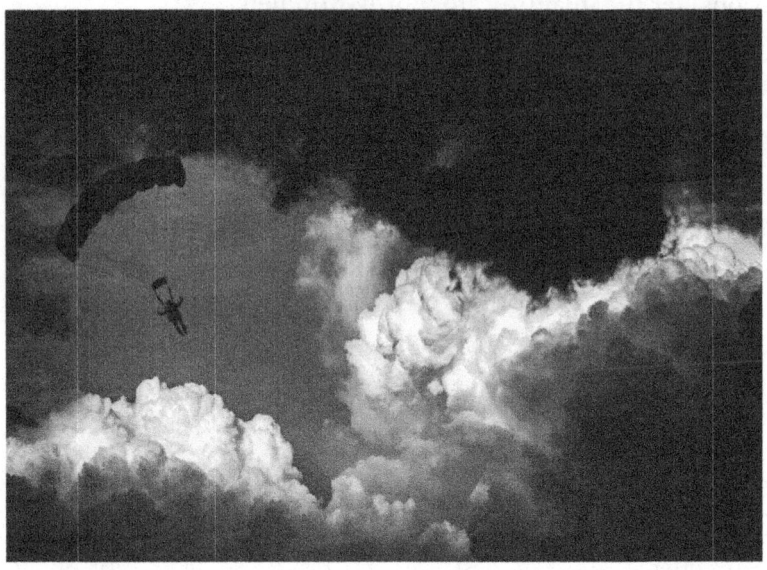

THE WAY TO VICTORY

1. Redefine Challenge

To turn problems into opportunities, most importantly, we'll need to change the way we define a problem. We'll need to see a problem as a form a challenge that will ultimately help us discover ourselves and grow our worth.

Instead of considering a problem as a nuisance, consider it as an opportunity to develop, to mature and to conquer ourselves. Remember, we always have to face stress and nuisances in life, one way or another. That's the intrinsic nature of life. Every one of us has to suffer sometimes. There's no exception to that.

As such, your capability to embrace and deal with challenges in life will determine your happiness and satisfaction. More than anything else. Eventually, we must step forward, confront and deal with our own challenges.

So the real questions are:

Can you embrace challenges and maintain a positive attitude?

Can you stop focusing on your negative thoughts and start thinking about a solution instead?

Can you move on and fight on relentlessly, even if your first solution failed?

Can you accept everything happened, embrace every mistake along the way, and consider other solutions to the problem?

Ultimately, the key is to **focus all your attention on finding solutions**, not on the negative feeling associated with the problem. To inspire yourself, you can use your imagination of success as a motivation to pull you forward. Imagine, when you're able to overcome those hardships and difficulties in life, how great will it be? How proud will you feel about yourself?

Imagine. And get excited when having an opportunity to face a problem in life. Because you're going to learn a lot, grow a lot, and eventually make it a better and worthier life.

One way or another, we can gradually find out our ways to take advantage of any problem. As we ponder upon the lessons that it brings, we can gain more experience and prevent similar events from happening in the future. Even better, we can develop our wisdom and courage through those hard times in life, thus feeling better and prouder about ourselves.

Extreme people who overcame extreme hardships and adversities in life don't see difficulties as mere troubles. They see difficulties as opportunities to prove themselves to the world. Instead of focusing their attention on the problem itself, they use the problem to learn necessary lessons, improve their strengths to bring happiness to themselves and others.

That is the way ultimate courage and strength can develop.

2. Take A Step Back To Have A Different View

When problems fall upon us, it's our tendency to stay trapped in the vicious cycle of stress and negativity, always asking ourselves self-defeating questions like "Why did this come to me?", "Why always me?"

It's very difficult to get out of this state if we don't take a step back and change our own perspective.

In fact, it's always easy to be obsessed with the flow of our negative thoughts in the midst of chaos. We therefore need to step back, calm down and regain our inner peace first. Self-awareness, deep breathing and meditation can help us achieve these important first steps.

Moreover, it's helpful to start asking ourselves proper questions. This is an important step in solving any problem we encounter in life.

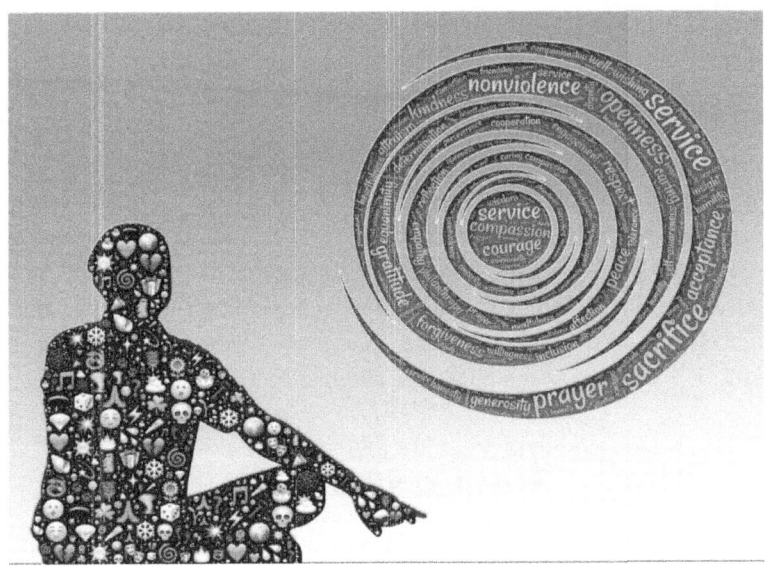

We can ask ourselves:

What problem is it?

On the scale of 1 to 10, how significant will it be after one year? Five years? And ten years?

Can I change the situation?

If no, then what lessons can I learn from this problem? How can I use it to grow myself and make my life better?

If yes, is it worth the effort to change the situation? Is it better that I just accept things as they are, or should I try to change things to make my life better?

What are the possible solutions to the problem? Is there anything new I haven't thought of?

Given this solution, what detailed plan and actions should I take? What can I use to motivate myself to take actions in a timely manner?

Who can help me with advices or help me carry out the actions? Who had similar problems in the past that I can consult or read about? How did they make it through? What detailed plan and mindset did they have?

As a matter of fact, it's highly likely that many people have experienced the same pain you're experiencing right now, and many of them could ultimately overcome it. As such, it's extremely helpful if you could learn from their struggles and victories. You'd be able to learn necessary skills, knowledge and attitude to confront the challenges yourself.

EMBRACE CHALLENGES

Challenges can only haunt us if we follow the flow of negative thinking and take no assessment. As we embrace each challenge, focus our effort on finding a solution and making ourselves better, challenges will then become our servants.

They don't control us anymore.

Instead, we'll control them all. We'll control what we think of the events, what we can learn from them, and what we'll do from this very moment onwards.

Thank you, challenges!

Thank you for giving me necessary skills and opportunities. Thank you for giving me the courage to move on and conquer my path.

From now on, I am the ultimate master of my way. I am the ultimate master of myself, my life, and my own happiness.

Thank You!

2

HOW TO ACCEPT THINGS THE WAY THEY ARE

Accept – then act. Whatever the present moment contains, accept it as if you had chosen it. Always work with it, not against it.

– **Eckhart Tolle**

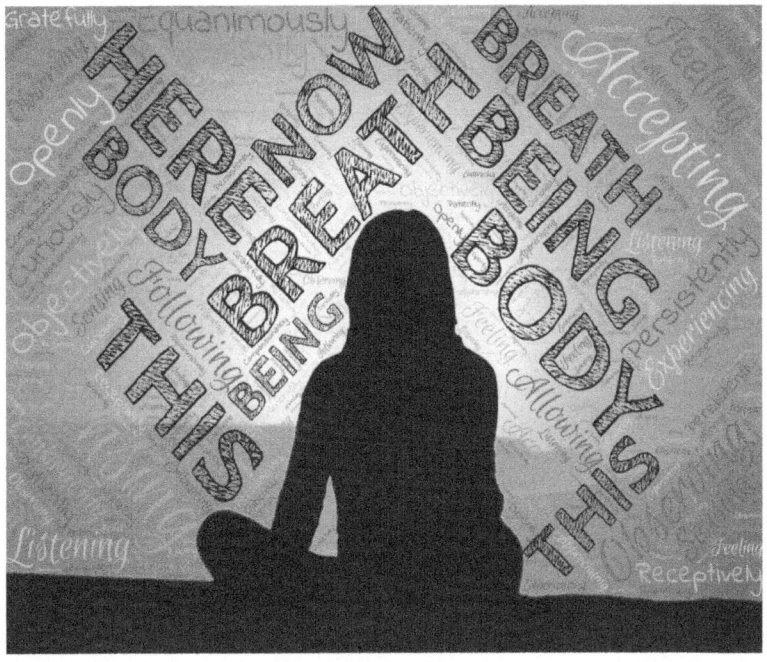

We always have to choose in life.

We can choose to fight against the world and its troubles. We can choose to focus on life's negative aspects and desperate to change other people. We can choose to obsess ourselves with the things that we don't have, and feel unhappy with the present as a result.

Or, we can choose to appreciate ourselves, everyone and everything around us. We can choose to be content with what we already have first, while constantly working our way to achieve better things. We can learn to accept and properly deal with everyone around first, before we can find those people that match us most.

In fact, embracing life as it is while working towards a better future is often the best remedy for fear, stress and anxiety.

This doesn't mean that we should always agree with someone or stay passive in every situation. This is to say that, instead, we should let go of the matters we can't control first. After that, we can take control by thinking about a detailed plan and then taking determined actions to carry out that plan.

The point is, when we cannot change a situation, it's time to change our mind.

It's time to accept and let go of the past, with its failures, agonies and losses.

It's time to accept the uncontrollable.

It's time to accept the unchangeable.

Learn the hard lessons.

And move on with the next plan in life.

That's the real meaning of acceptance.

THE POWER OF ACCEPTANCE

Since a few years ago I have learned the great power of acceptance.

For example, I usually hated the weather when it came to winter. I disliked the bitter cold temperature that caused me so much discomfort. As it eventually turned out, it was actually my point of view that brought me stress and worries in small situations like that.

Again, it's a choice I had to make.

The realization was that I couldn't do anything except adapting to the weather, finding exciting activities and enjoying it. Accepting the weather and learning to live with it was the only good choice I had. The other choice was to complain about the weather and suffer from the severe stress of that constant struggle.

I realized that I was much more peaceful and cheerful when I accepted what life had given me, instead of continually struggling to control everything.

Acceptance is being comfortable with what we're given. It is improving changeable aspects of our life, and embracing the unchangeable ones. It means letting go of the things we cannot control while staying active on the matters that we can deal with. Whether it's a terminal disease, a tragic accident, a sudden loss of someone we love, accepting things that we cannot control will help us stay in peace. Practicing acceptance will help us move on despite the unexpected ups and downs of life, in the moments that we're uncertain of what's going to fall upon us next.

There are often times we're alone in life. Everyone else is busy with their life, with their own stress, hassles and anxiety. No one really cares about us, about our worries and depression. No one has spare time to care about our sadness or loneliness. As such, during those difficult times, it's ourselves and ourselves alone that we can rely upon. That's what we must accept to be a strong and independent person.

Furthermore, when facing with a gloomy reality, with painful and depressing matters, we've got to recognize that not everything in life can always be the way we want it to be. If we cannot change a situation, then it's best that we learn to accept it. It's best to embrace and go with the flow of life instead of struggling with uncontrollable disturbances that fall upon us.

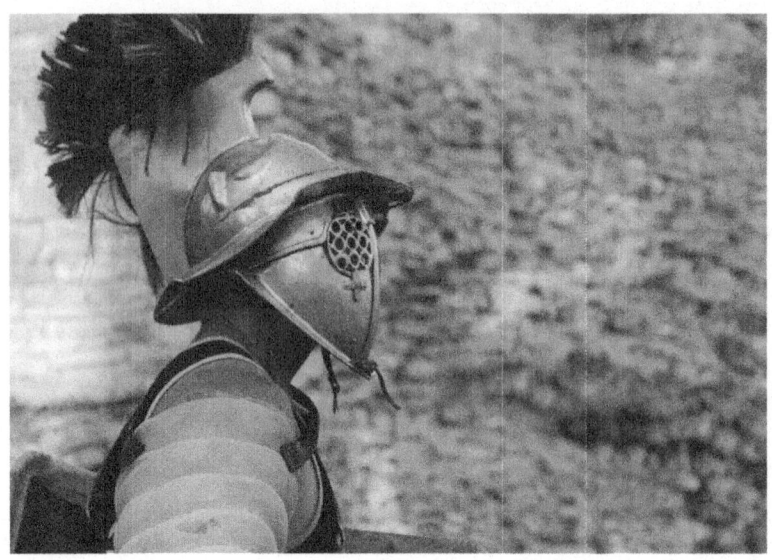

LEANRING TO ACCEPT

Learning to accept those aspects of life that we cannot change is a vital skill. Doing so will help us alleviate all burdens and be truly liberated.

Most of us want to possess many things in life. We want everything to be perfect. Truth is, that desire of perfection is often the ultimate source of our miseries. Life is so much paradoxical - the more you want to control it, the more you are controlled and burdened. The more you want to possess, the more stress and fear of losses you'll have to overcome.

On the contrary, the less you expect from life, the less troubling and painful you'll fight against it. And of course, the more fulfilling your life will become.

We hence need to accept and let go of unchangeable things.

Accept death. Everyone has to face death eventually, one way or another. So while we feel sad after the loss of someone we love, remind ourselves that death is an unchangeable part of life. It is indeed inevitable. Remind ourselves that maybe, we would ultimately join everyone we love in the afterlife. As such, do our best to make this life the most unforgettable one, so that we can share many wonderful stories to our beloved ones when we meet them in the future.

Accept negative emotions. Accept that life can be boring, brutal or difficult sometimes. Accept that we will fail times and times again. Every one of us exists for a different reason, so we don't need to gain glorious achievements to be valuable or worthy in life. As long as we treat others kindly, do our best, and have some inspiring dreams to strive for in life, we can march on to happiness with our heads held high.

Also, embrace your imperfections. Many people wish for a perfect family, a perfect body, or a perfect partner in life. But there is no perfect family. There is no perfect partner. And there is no perfect life. Everything has both positive and negative aspects associated with it. In reality, almost no one can find their perfect imaginations. The mere fantasy of perfection might even create cracks in our relationships, when our expectations exceed what we can get from reality.

Instead, learn to accept our flaws as well as others'. Reconsider our improper expectations. Relationships are always two-way streets that need cooperation and effort from both sides. A great relationship is not something that we can find. It's something you and your partner must create together.

A NEW LIFE HAS COME

To get out of all troubles, first we need to take a step back. We need to gradually accept every mistake, every hardship and every failure in life. Life is here for us to learn and grow from our mistakes. So take it as a game, and only a game - an exciting one in which hardships are merely necessary challenges for us to level up. It is a game that we need to decide what's controllable and what's not, what we can learn from each trouble, and what's the best thing to do right now.

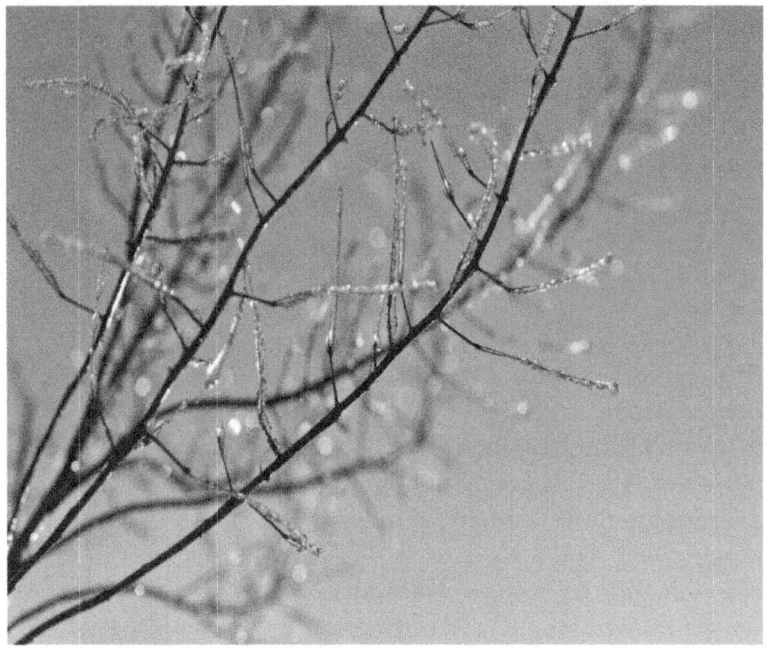

After all, no one can be successful without those difficult moments of hardships and adversities. I haven't seen one. Have you?

Eventually, nothing lasts forever. We can only stay young and vibrant for a certain stage of life. After that, we'll get old. We'll get sick. Each of us passes through various periods of life. We may stay intoxicated in love, lose ourselves in romance, build our family, and finally lose the one we love. Live and die. Life and death. We're all the same.

Remember, everyone will live, love, succeed, blunder and eventually say goodbye. No exception. The important thing is, we can learn to embrace it all. We can learn to feel grateful for this chance to breathe and discover this world. We can then get excited and appreciate our privilege to participate in Life.

Indeed, if something lasts forever, it's not something special any more. Death, as negative as it seems, is the exact thing that makes every living moment valuable.

Normally, it happens that we humans often desire superficial things. We want more. More. And more. The question is, why do we have to burden ourselves with so many desires? Isn't it better that we learn to accept, forgive, and embrace life as it is now? Many people can live happily without being rich, without having a family, falling in love or having an intact body.

So why can't we?

Indeed, the key for happiness is to genuinely appreciate what we're given, while accepting that we cannot have everything in life. That's how we let ourselves be free and truly joyful.

After all, life is meant to give us challenges so that we can stumble, rise up and then grow. Life is meant to be accepted and forgiven for whatever happened. Acceptance is not weakness. Acceptance is power. Acceptance is the ultimate key to a happy and fulfilling life. Acceptance is what gives us a better future and a better opportunity.

Then inner peace will be within our hand.

3

THE MOST IMPORTANT LOVE

You've got to love yourself first. You've got to be okay on your own before you can be okay with somebody else.

- Jennifer Lopez

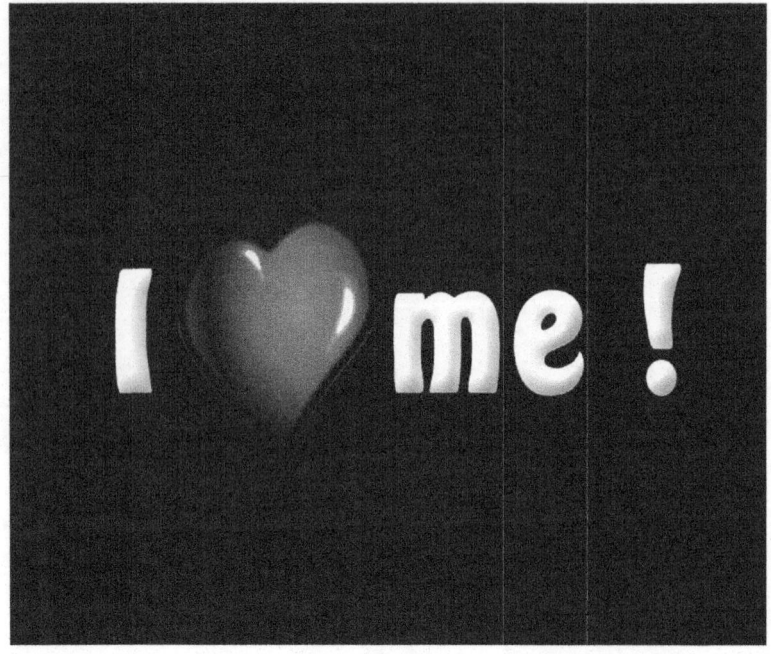

Are you loving yourself the right way?

Almost everyone understands how to love someone else. We spend so much time to find love and give love to other people.

But how about giving love to one's self?

Do you love yourself enough?

Loving one's self is an unfamiliar notion to many people. Loving yourself is the respect, kindness and acceptance you give to yourself. It's the recognition that you deserve to be respected and appreciated by other people. It's the positive attitude that you have about yourself and your life.

Eventually, your life quality depends on two things: how you view yourself, and how you view the world and other people. Having a positive view about yourself is the first and also a critical step that contributes to your long-term happiness.

When you love yourself, you're able to recognize your positive aspects and embrace your imperfect ones, thereby improving your self-esteem. Loving yourself also facilitates your interaction with the outside world and gives you a better perspective of it. Loving yourself is thus the secret to any long-term independence and fulfillment in life.

THE MEANING OF SELF-LOVE

Self-love is the unconditional love, the total respect and acceptance you have for your own self. It means that no matter how many failures and mistakes you've made, you can still accept yourself and find some ways to improve it. It means that no matter how bad and how sad life has been sometimes, you can still give yourself another chance to work towards a better future.

Eventually, you don't need to beat yourself up for what was

wrong. Instead, you can learn to let your soul be filled with healing, acceptance, and love.

Loving yourself is to **rely on your strength** against any negative event that happens. It means that you don't let yourself to be primarily dependent on the outside environment. It means that you know how to enjoy your days even if you are alone in life. And even if this whole world crumbles, you can still bounce back and find your way to love.

Loving yourself is to **recognize your value and efforts in life**. It means that you are truly proud of what you've achieved so far. That you truly appreciate your life without needing anyone to understand, praise or validate your worth. You yourself are enough for appreciating your value in this world.

Loving yourself is to **understand your shortcomings and be comfortable with them**. It means to fall in love with your real self, even it's full of mistakes and shortcomings. It means to love the unique differences that make you who you are. After all, everyone has his own weaknesses and imperfections. And weaknesses help define his unique existence in life. So, the most important thing we need to do is to accept ourselves. Only after that can we try our best to improve, grow and succeed each day.

Loving yourself is to **feel okay with yourself and with whatever you have in hands**. It means that you don't have to compare yourself with anyone else, because you understand that everyone of us is unique in our own way. You can feel content with whatever you're given in life, in knowing that you can always work harder to make your life even better.

Loving yourself is to **have clear boundaries in your relationships**. It means that you don't allow other people to cross the boundaries and hurt you in life. It means that although you're willing to listen to other people's opinions, you don't let anyone control what you do. And if you feel that a relationship is toxic or harmful, you're willing to walk away with no regret.

WHY SELF-LOVE?

Why is loving yourself important?

When you love yourself the right way, you'll be able to recognize your own values and positive aspects. You'll feel confident and have a healthy self-esteem. And even if disasters strike, you can still rely on yourself to regain happiness.

When you love yourself, you'll be able to understand who you are, what suits you and what doesn't. You can connect to your soul and live with its inner peace. You'll be able to tap into your inner courage and strength to face every hardship in life.

When you love yourself, you'll learn to love others in a proper way. You'll learn to establish clear responsibilities by setting what you accept and what you don't. You'll be able to communicate clearly and let others know what you're unhappy about. You won't need to impress or seek for the validation from anyone. You'll be able to appreciate people who support you, and leave any toxic relationship that's damaging your life.

When you love yourself, you'll be able to control your direction in life. You'll learn to rely less on other people for your own happiness. You'll be able to rely on yourself for your life's satisfaction instead. You'll learn to take responsibility for everything happens, and take control of what you think and do.

In fact, if you don't love yourself enough, no one in this world can give you the self-esteem and satisfaction you wish. When you don't love yourself enough, you'll put a lot of expectations on other people and the outside world. You'll rely on them for your own happiness. That's a huge mistake, in fact, because those emotions always come and leave very quickly.

Eventually, you can't control other people and much of the

outside world. Sooner or later they'll go against your expectations. And if you always rely on them, you'll feel hurt. That's the reason why you should look for your own happiness from the inside. That's why you should love yourself and rely on yourself during difficult times in life. This kind of inner love and appreciation is your eternal power, and no one can ever take it away from you.

Loving oneself is thus critical. That said, that's not an easy task at all, especially for people who often act based on the expectations of others. In these cases, it's easy for a person to forget his own needs and criticize himself for even small mistakes.

There are usually several reasons for this.

Negativity bias

Imagine there's one person who praises you and what you're doing, who tells you that you are kind and talented, that you're contributing to make this life better. This person likes you and encourages other people to follow your example.

Now imagine that there's another person who just does the opposite. He thinks you're a lazy, stupid and impolite person. He dislikes you and always disclaims others from making friends with you.

Which person will get more of your attention?

In reality, most of us will be much more obsessed with the second person. This is what we call "negativity bias", which is our mental tendency to focus on the negative sides of ourselves and the outside world. It causes us to feel bad not only about ourselves and our lives, but also about the world and other people around us. We are unfortunately wired to be more sensitive to negative aspects of everything.

Media's effect

This is another major reason why loving yourself is difficult.

Every day, we are continually bombarded with thousands of stories of successful people. They appear everywhere on media. They're praised, admired and adored by millions of others. The widespread power of media eventually leads us to doubt ourselves. We start to see ourselves as someone ugly, incompetent and useless.

Under the effect of media, loving yourself is just too difficult.

In reality, those famous and successful people are just the minorities. Most of us are actually ordinary people having our own normal lives. That said, an ordinary life can still be a happy, fulfilling and meaningful one, as long as we have a burning purpose and a clear direction to follow.

HOW TO LOVE YOURSELF

1. Recognize Your Worth

Recall your past achievements, no matter how small they were.

Think of the things you have that many others don't.

Recall some moments in life when you helped people or made their lives better.

Truth is, every one of us has our own strengths and weaknesses. As such, it's not necessary to merely focus on your negative qualities.

Instead, begin to appreciate your positive aspects. And be proud of them! Write down a list of 5 aspects that you love about yourself. And renew it every day.

Along your path, start celebrating and feeling proud about yourself whenever you help people or achieve something. These moments of celebrations would help you enhance your self-esteem and happiness in life. The road to self-love often begins with small steps that gradually turn into regular habits.

2. Take It Easy On Yourself

Every one of us has many weaknesses. Every one of us has made many mistakes in life. So, take it easy on your mistakes and weaknesses.

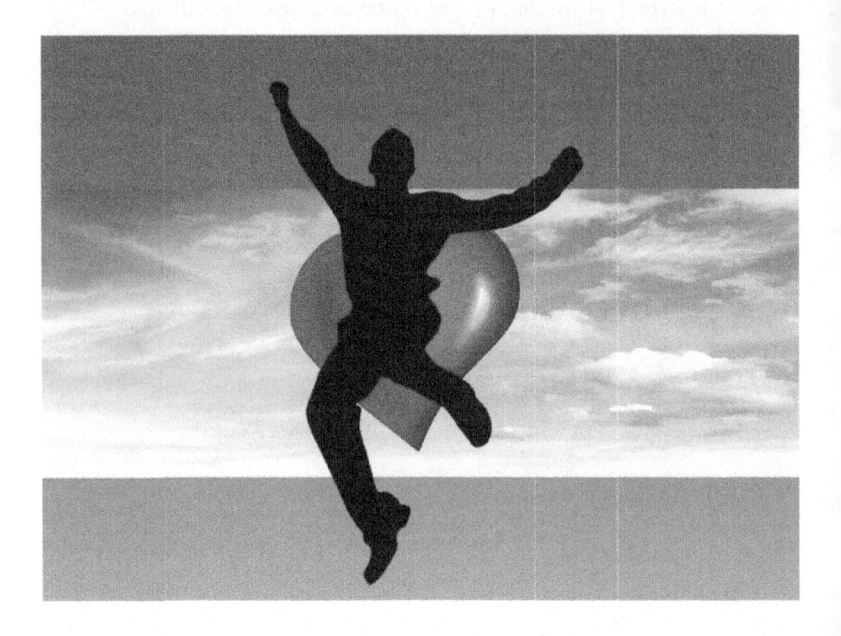

And don't be obsessed with the way you look. When you love yourself, you won't need to care so much about that anymore. Because after all, appearance is just a small part of you. Besides appearance, you also have your soul, your kindness, courage, your work, family and friends who support you. Appearance is not primarily who you are. It's not everything in life. It doesn't determine how worthy or how helpful a person you can be.

Appearance is only important under the influence of media and naive thinking.

After all, do the people who truly care about you do so just because of how you look?

Remember, it's always better to focus on your pride and self-love. If you want an everlasting love, it's the kind of love that always resides inside yourself. You just need to explore your soul and do whatever you're passionate about. And take it easy if you make some mistakes. After all, you can always grow and make yourself better. That's what truly matters!

3. Set Clear Boundaries

In reality, it's not helpful to always play it safe and agree with everyone's ideas. Instead, voice your own thoughts and expectations to other people. Allow yourself to say no when you feel you don't want to follow the way other people expect you to be.

Moreover, always consider if some relationships are truly good for you. If a relationship turns out to be harmful, allow yourself to leave it without any regret or hesitation. Setting clear boundaries of what you can and what you can't accept will bring you healthy and meaningful relationships in life.

In addition, take your time to find people who like you for who you are. Take your time to find your tribe. Spending time with people you like and having mutual support is a great way to take care of yourself.

4. Have A Date

Eventually, we can't rely on others for an everlasting love. It's because most outside factors are constantly changing, and we can never make them to be like what we wish. Romantic love is great, but it is meaningless without our ability to be independent and comfortable with ourselves. Self-love is the ultimate source of every kind of affection.

As such, why don't we now bring a great life to ourselves first?

Today, you can have a date with yourself. Treat yourself like your beloved lover. Take a deep breath. Go out for a great meal. Have a healthy drink. Enjoy your favorite music. And do something you like.

Today, be your own lover. Don't wait for anyone else to give you the best gifts and experiences in life. You must do that for yourself. Right now!

Cause this is ultimately your life. Not anyone else's.

5. Forgive Yourself

Remember that everyone has made many mistakes in life. And that's okay. As often, we tend to be more sympathetic towards other people than towards ourselves. To have a great path in life, therefore, it's important to erase any negative self-image and turn your attention to a positive one.

When you face a problem in life, imagine how you would talk to a friend facing the same dilemma. Treat yourself like that.

And always be compassionate with yourself. It's important to recognize your inner critical voice and stop them from growing.

Consider these situations:

When you look into the mirror

When you get angry

When you are insulted by someone

When you increase weight

When you make mistakes in life

When you lie to someone

When you are lazy

When you smoke

When you enjoy harmful foods and drink

When you don't do exercises

When someone you love doesn't love you

When your expectations are not met.

Do you still love yourself in these situations? And what do you often tell yourself then? If it's negative and critical, you'll need to erase your inner critic.

Sometimes, what you judge about yourself might reside inside your head all the time, without you even being aware of them. The longer and the more often you have those thoughts, the firmer a belief they'll become. As such, it's important to stop those negative thoughts and replace them with positive ones. Not easy. But you can do that gradually and improve your self-image each day.

So, the next time that you catch yourself being self-critical, stop it. Immediately! Instead, tell yourself something more supportive and encouraging. For example, you can tell yourself, "I can learn from this situation and avoid it in the future", "I can start again from where I stumbled", "Success is not how many achievements I've had, it's how many times I fall down and stand up again!"

After that, start planning and doing what you need to do.

Truth is, after being self-critical for a long time, sometimes it's hard to sympathize with yourself. If so, it's helpful to imagine that you are a little child. You look lovely, sensitive, and need a lot of support from other people. You often fail or make mistakes, but it's understandable because you can always learn more and grow more from that.

6. Let Go Of The Past

In order to love ourselves, we need to be detached from our past pains and experiences. Usually, we let those stressful events haunt our soul and break our heart, even if they were really long gone. We often allow them to affect our emotions, confidence and quality of life.

In reality, each of us was let down sometimes. Each of us was hurt badly, one way or another. Each of us has experienced sadness, frustration, sorrow and anger in life. Each of us has had wounds, aches and scars all over our heart.

That said, the past doesn't exist anymore. The past merely exists inside our mind in the form of memories. Eventually, how much the past can traumatize us depends on how much we let it linger on. It depends on how much we focus our attention on the long gone past instead of enjoying this precious present.

To reach for a happier and more fulfilling life, we need to let go. We need to live in this present. We need to move forward. Relentlessly.

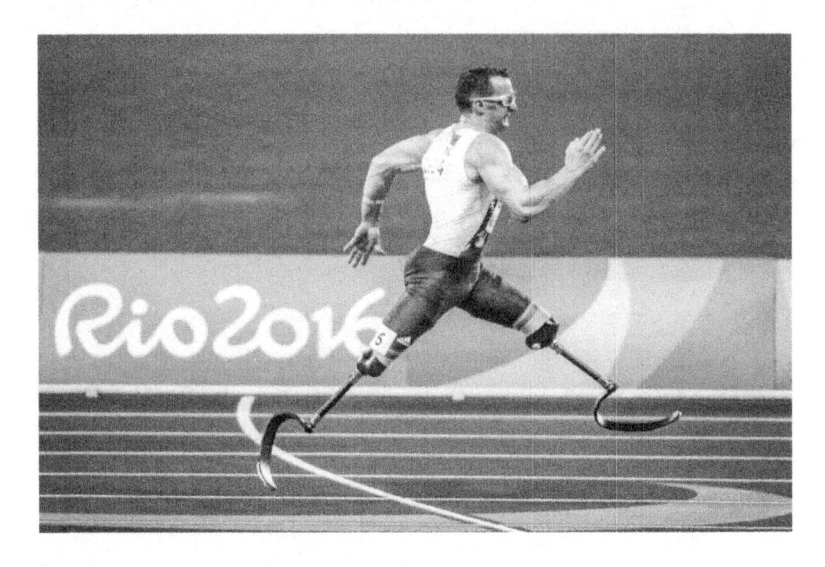

7. Take Care Of Your Health

To achieve a fulfilling life, it's vital to take care of your health. Ultimately, your health can affect your energy, emotions and quality of life directly. It's in fact much more important than how you look on the outside.

Today, start taking good care of yourself. Start eating fruits and vegetables regularly. Avoid consuming too much fast foods and sugary drinks. Go to bed early. Do regular exercises. Sit under the sun. Read your favorite books. Enjoy the beauty of nature. And sing a song you love.

Today, take a great care of yourself. Like nothing else matters more.

Today, let everyone around be envied with your inner fire. Let you yourself glow with love and confidence.

8. Stop Comparing Yourself With Others

As often, we tend to forget our good qualities and merely focus on what we don't have. For example, while being single we tend to compare ourselves with people who are in a long-term relationship. But many of them are probably looking at us and wishing that they were as free and independent.

The grass always seems to be greener on the other side. But that's not necessarily true.

Remember, each of us has our own clock. We don't need to live like anyone else and make it all a race. Instead, we can take our time to enjoy what we do have in hands, while planning and taking actions to improve our future. We can appreciate beautiful aspects of our life, while gradually growing and improving ourselves to make it even better.

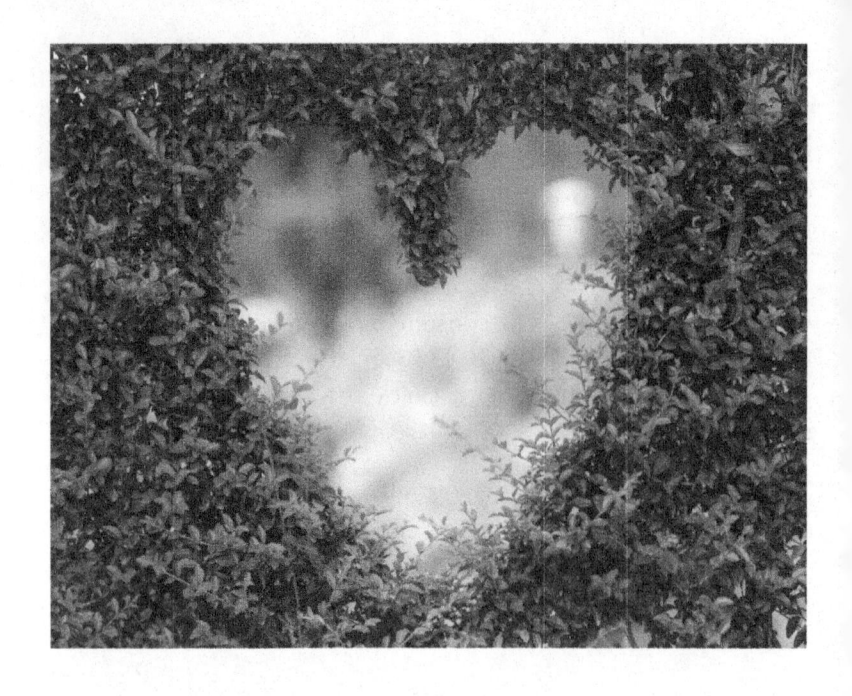

YOU YOURSELF ARE THE MOST IMPORTANT PERSON

Life is a journey of self-discovery. It's a journey to explore who we are and what kind of beauty is lying inside us. It's a journey to make ourselves and the world around a better place. To be able to embark on such an enduring and wonderful journey, therefore, you'll need to take good care of yourself, body and soul. You'll need to make that a major priority. Above everything else.

Loving yourself is about appreciating yourself for who you are, for all of your strengths and weaknesses. It's about forgiving your own failures and mistakes, letting go of the pains of the past, and marching heroically to create a better future.

You can choose to rely on yourself or the outside environment for your own happiness. You can choose to determine your own worth or depend on the judgement of others. You can choose to forgive yourself or become your worst critic. You can choose to live with love, gratitude and mindfulness, or without them all.

What do you choose?

4

DETACHING FROM NEGATIVE FEELINGS

Detachment doesn't mean I'm trying less hard. It just means that fears and emotions that used to torment and paralyze me longer have the same power over me.

- **Kelly Cultrone**

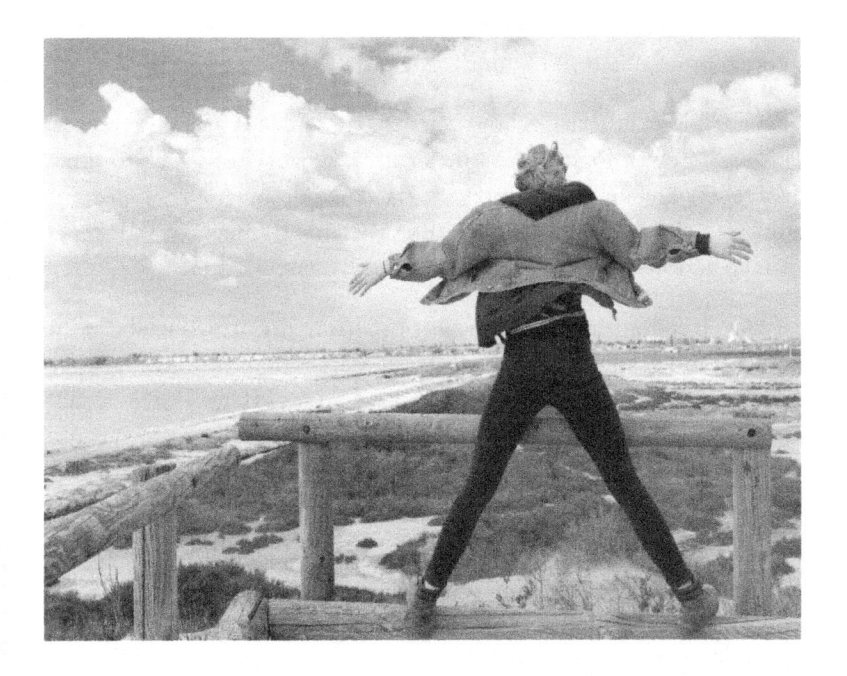

Many of us have been told to follow our heart.

Sounds reasonable. Because listening to our heart can sometimes help us make quick decisions in urgent situations.

But it's not always a good idea to listen to one's heart. Many people who rely on their emotions often make terrible mistakes and eventually lead to major disasters.

The problem is that feelings themselves are not usually correct. Feelings are not logical. And they can be wrong from time to time. In reality, feelings could prevent us from doing many important things that we need to do. On the other hand, they can induce us to take actions that are harmful to ourselves and others.

In fact, trusting our feelings can obscure us from taking the right actions and lead us the wrong way. Very often, gloomy feelings trap us in the cycle of blaming and negativity. If we don't detach from those feelings and take necessary actions to improve the situation, things can always go worse. Always listening to our heart will thus cause ultimate destruction and stagnation to our lives.

Emotions are usually wrong for you.

For example, you might be aware that consuming fast foods regularly or having no exercises is harmful to your health. However, you usually cannot stop eating or being lazy. The temptation of having a good feeling is too powerful. Against all logic, you let yourself be trapped in the gradual destruction of life.

Maybe you know that you need to leave a toxic relationship to free yourself, but you still cling on that relationship and let it ruin your soul. You still hope the person would change and tolerate his bad behaviors times after times.

Maybe you know that you should work harder to achieve success in life, but you're overwhelmed by emotions and procrastination that you can't find any motivation to make a start.

WHY CAN'T WE TRUST OUR FEELINGS

Feelings are unreliable. As often, there are many feelings that come up in our minds. They are signals for us to change some aspects of life and make it better. However, our actions need to be pondered upon carefully. Acting impulsively based on pure emotions is extremely harmful, especially when it comes to strong emotions like anger, stress, anxiety and depression.

There are the reasons why feelings are unreliable:

Feelings Are Not Accurate

Feelings are not logical. They are created by our instincts, thoughts and experiences. So although feelings can act as signals to inform us about a problem that's going on, these signals can be too extreme or inappropriate. As such, feelings are not always true. Feeling bad about yourself doesn't mean you are truly bad. Feeling good while watching TV doesn't mean you should continue to do so. Feeling someone is the right person for you doesn't mean that's exactly the truth.

So instead of always following your heart, take a step back. Breathe. And let yourself be calm. After that, explore the facts underneath your feelings. See whether they are true facts or not. Find out the origins of those thoughts and feelings.

The key here is to be proactive instead of being reactive to the situation and its associated feelings. In order to make a good plan and find a way out, you'll need to rely on facts and logic, not emotions.

Feelings Are Not Who You Are

Feelings are merely a portion of you. Because apart from your feelings, you also have your body and soul. As such, your feelings are not everything you have. It's not entirely who you are in this world.

So, don't take your feelings like it's your whole self. Maybe you often have negative feelings. Maybe you often feel bad about yourself and your own life. But those bad feelings don't necessarily imply that you are bad. They don't necessarily imply that you are not worthy.

You are your own spirit. You are your own soul. Each and every soul is valuable. And you can make yourself worthy in spite of any negative feeling or situation you've experienced.

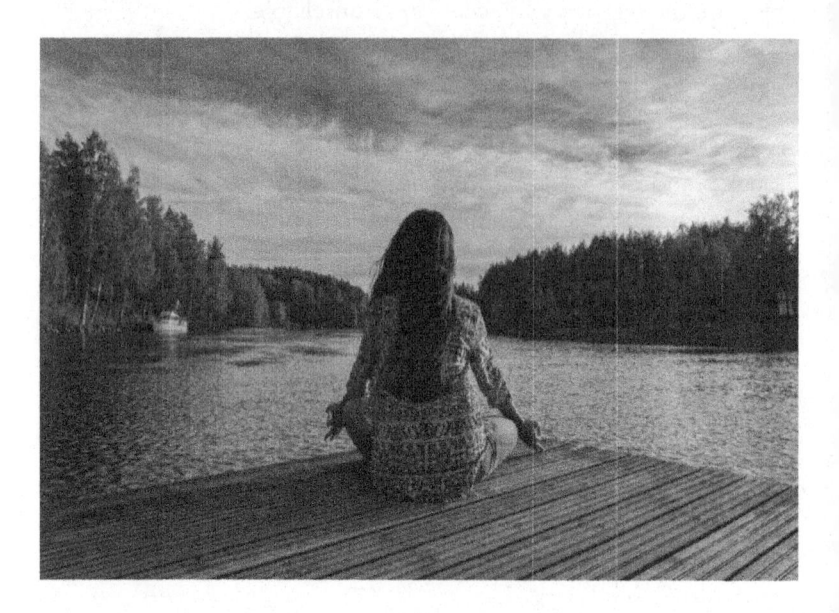

Feelings Are Short-Term

Feelings don't last forever. They come and then go away. They flow in and then they flow out of our mind. As a matter of fact, the more we accept and find comfort with that constant flow, the more peaceful we'll get. The more we resist and fight against our feelings, the more difficult our life will become.

If there's any negativity going on, take a step back. Close your eyes. Take some deep breaths. Accept the present feeling. Then find something meaningful to do and focus on it instead. In knowing for sure that, this bad feeling does not necessarily mean anything. It's just a temporary phenomenon. And it will go away really soon.

WHAT TO DO WITH FEELINGS, THEN?

If you think that strong feelings often cause troubles for you in life, it's time to ponder upon the matter and learn to deal with your feelings.

Most of the time, a feeling occurs due to your expectations. If reality is similar or above your expectations, you're likely to feel good. Otherwise, you'll feel bad about the situation.

It's important to recognize that your feelings merely act as signals of your expectations for life. Appreciate them for that. But nothing more. Your feelings don't show what's real in the world. A wonderful life for one person might seem to be too boring for another one. Similar events could cause different feelings in different people. These different feelings come from different perspectives and different expectations. That's what feelings are all about.

So begin to appreciate your feelings for showing you how much your inner world and the outer world fit together. But don't let feelings enslave you. For example, feeling bad about yourself and your life doesn't necessarily mean that you are bad. On the other hand, feeling good about someone or something doesn't always mean that you should attach yourself to that person or that thing at all cost.

Embrace and accept your feelings, but remind yourself that that they don't necessarily reflect any reality, and they will definitely not last forever.

Moreover, it's important to stop having any immediate response to your feelings. Feelings are not a logical process, thus they can lead you to the wrong actions and directions in life. As such, it's often better to take a step back, calm yourself down, and analyze the situation first.

Instead of succumbing to the feeling of low self-esteem or inadequacy, you can now accept that feeling and march on in spite of it. Because you know that you can always think of a plan to make life better.

Instead of surrendering yourself to the feeling of being lazy and postponing your work, you can now ignore that feeling and start working now.

Instead of letting your anger or anxiety control how you behave, you can now sit back and think of some ways to solve all troubling matters.

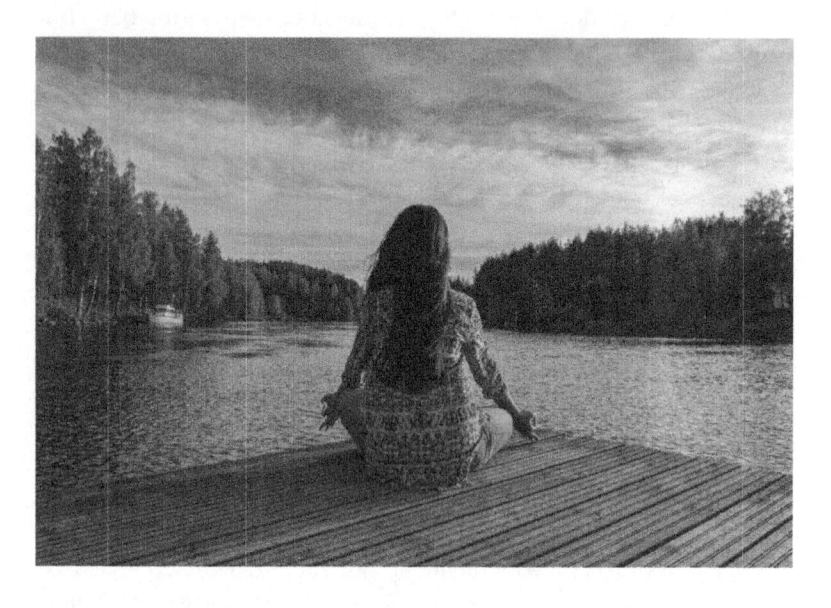

EVERYTHING WILL PASS

Emotions are usually wrong. Hence, stop making decisions based on your emotions. For example, when it's necessary to punish a disrespectful behavior or discard a toxic relationship, go ahead to do so even if you don't want to. Base your actions on logic, on the consideration of all pros and cons of the situation instead. That way, you'll find your peace and success in life.

Also, it's important to be aware of your toxic desire for perfection in life, which could usually cause you to feel inadequate about your life and yourself. As often, we tend to focus on our shortcomings and forget about our positive aspects. This tendency usually creates a low self-esteem and a variety of negative feelings. Instead of surrendering to that tendency, now you can learn to focus on your positive qualities, on how kindly you've helped others, how hard-working you've been, or how courageous you've overcome great hardships and difficulties in life.

Remember, no matter how bad your life has been, there are always people out there with much worse situations. Yet, many can still fight on and succeed despite going through so much blood and pains in life.

Also, in order to be more successful, you will need to push yourself beyond your procrastination and comfort zone. Do something. And do it now! Don't wait until tomorrow. Don't wait until you get the motivation. Because it will hardly come. Instead, employ the mindset of "Everything important must get started today!"

Be bold. Be relentless. Because you know how great your life will be in the long term if you start working today. Because you know that if you don't, you may get some short-term comfort but will regret a lot later in life.

So today, at this very moment, you can start. Start defeating all procrastination. Start detaching from your feelings, and actively planning your life instead. Start working and walking towards your ultimate dreams.

Always keep in mind that feelings are not who you are. Feelings can always be changed by your thoughts and your actions. Feelings are trivial. It's your soul and your actions that matter more.

Accept your feelings. Just let them come and go away.

Remember, they all will pass.

5

THE CURE OF DESIRES

Gratitude is the healthiest of all human emotions. The more you express gratitude for what you have, the more likely you will have even more to express gratitude for.

- Zig Ziglar

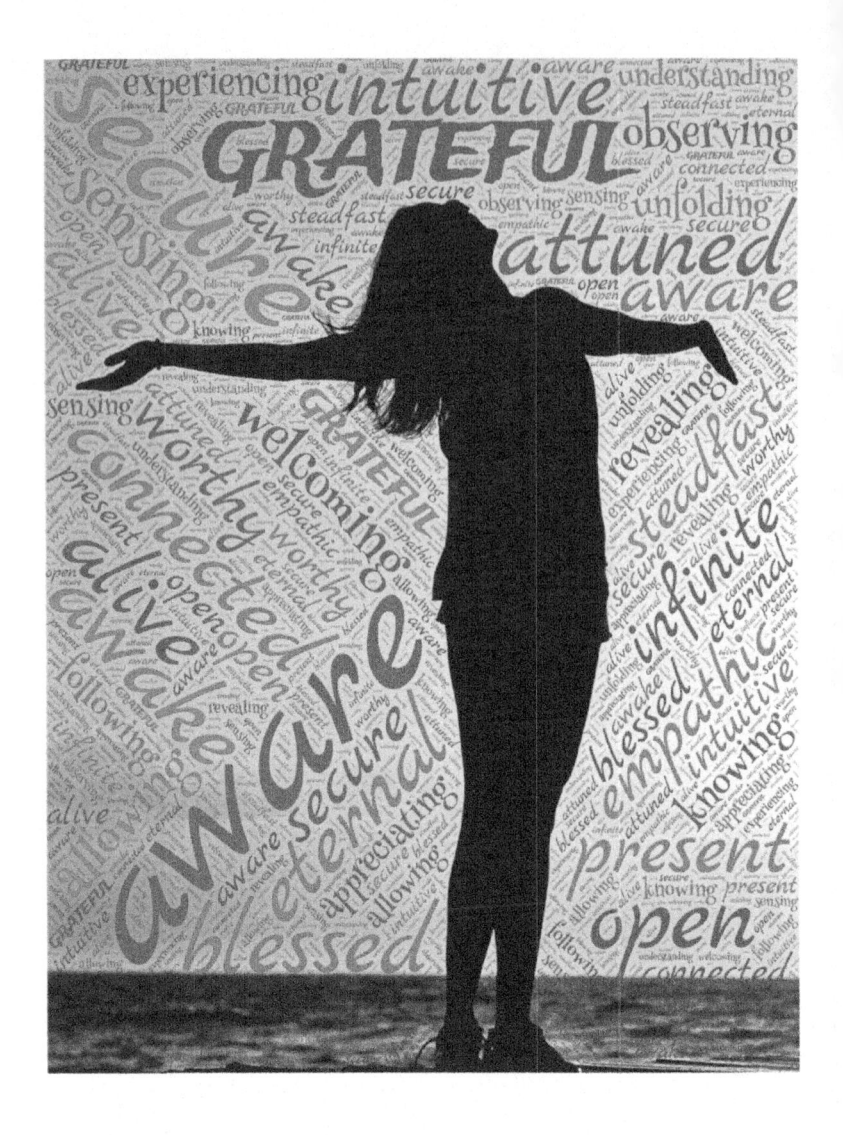

Do you often have many complaints,

Compare yourself with other people,

And obsess your mind with something you can't get?

As often, life bombards us with various unexpected situations and difficulties. As that happens, we tend to blame and complain about our lives. Complaining and desiring are often a part of our daily behavior, a vicious trap that we easily fall into.

Truth is, while it's sometimes healthy to wish for something and take effort to actively achieve it, merely obsessing our minds with desires and complaints is ultimately a recipe for unhappiness and dissatisfaction. It is often a source of constant stress and headaches.

Eventually, our headaches come because we often ignore or underestimate what we do have in life, and at the same time focus so much on what we don't have. They come because we fantasize about the things that we can't get. We're obsessed with how great our lives would be if we had them in life. We tend to overestimate the pleasure that our dreams bring about, and underestimate the problems associated with the things that we wish for.

For example, we often fantasize about the joy of material success. We tend to get obsessed with getting rich. We tend to ignore all possible pains and sacrifices needed to reach for it: time, peace, health, family and friendship, just to name a few. As such, the obsession will cease as soon as we start focusing on the fantasy's negative aspects, as well as appreciating the importance of various blessings we're already given.

We also fantasize about the sweetness of romance. We tend to forget all possible conflicts, quarrels, pains and problems associated with it. Maybe falling in love wouldn't make you feel better, but instead would create more struggles and headaches in life.

As a matter of fact, we tend to forget and underestimate those people and things that we already have in life. We tend to overestimate and dream about what we don't possess. It's all about appreciation and imagination. It's all about our instinct which gradually habituates ourselves to the old pleasures, at the same time desires and searches for newer ones.

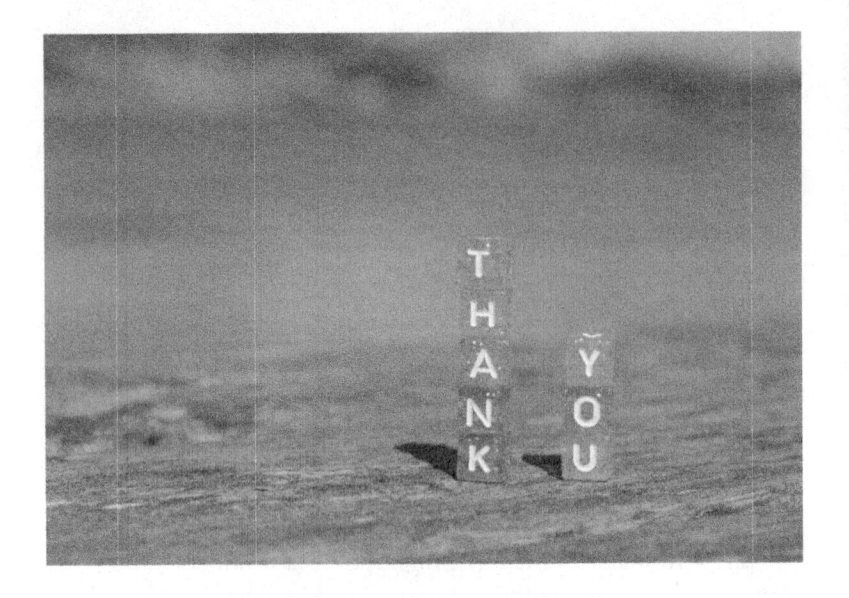

What's more, our headaches come because we don't have clear priorities in life. We have a lengthy wish list of getting rich, being healthy, lively, successful and beautiful, among many others. We desire so many things and wish for so many wins in life. We obsess our soul with almost everything we could imagine.

That said, it's impossible to achieve it all. A rich businessman may not have much time taking care for his own family. A famous celebrity may have been enduring traumatic pains with his romantic life. A good-looking person may find himself short of knowledge and skills. In fact, it usually happens that we cannot achieve everything we want. And refusing to accept this fact would be a great source of dissatisfaction in life.

GETTING OUT OF TROUBLES

As often, various problems keep disrupting our tranquility and obsessing our mind. The more we think about them, the more we'll keep focusing on their negative aspects, and eventually we'll be trapped in a cycle of negativity.

How can we escape from this vicious cycle?

Normally, the problem is reduced as we learn to **appreciate life** more. It diminishes as we remind ourselves that our lives will end soon, and that everything will eventually be lost. We indeed possess nothing in the long term. We possess nothing at all to fear losses or worries. And one day, we will turn into dust and oblivion. All of us.

Being aware of our end, we can then live and love without any doubt or fear. We can then stop wishing for more, more, and more. We can then be thankful for the life we're given today.

Come what may.

The problem is also reduced as we **let go of the need to control** the world around. It diminishes as we abandon the thoughts of how external matters and how our own lives should be.

It goes away as we learn to love the life we have, and wholeheartedly embrace it. No matter what happened along our way.

The problem is reduced as we **set clear priorities** in life. It fades away as we identify which is necessary and which is not, at this very moment. It fades away when we focus on our major priorities, and at the same time temporarily ignore minor ones for the current period of life.

In fact, we need to understand that we can't have everything we wish. We need to acknowledge that it's natural to be imperfect, one way or another. And then realize that it's totally okay to lack many things we want. Keep in mind that we can always appreciate and enjoy what we have in hand first, before we can make a plan and strive for more ambitious goals in life.

The problem is also reduced as we **acknowledge positive things around us**. It diminishes as we stop focusing on negative aspects of our lives and the world around. Stress and worries, anxieties and distress, regrets and pains, we all experience them from time to time. But it's up to us to decide whether we let them linger on our mind, or we accept and let go of their shackles. It's a vital choice that we all have to make.

For now, try to recall your great moments of joy, excitement, happiness and thankfulness in life. Recall those moments in which you were living truly and fully. Then list 3 things that you're grateful for. And send thanks to all supportive people and positive things that came into your life.

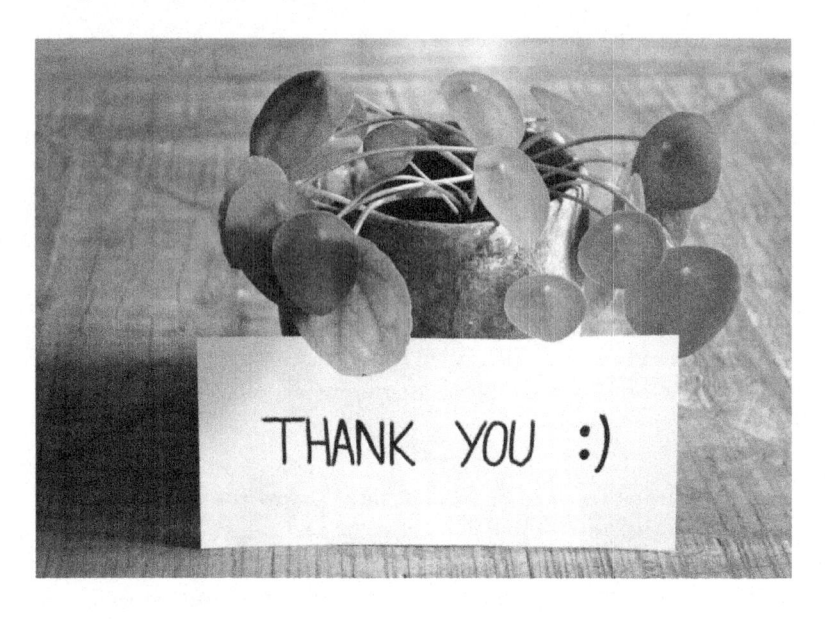

The problem is furthermore reduced as we step outside ourselves and **look at many lives that are much worse than ours**. It diminishes as we look at things from a grander perspective, as we look at those extreme hardships that many people have to endure that we could never have imagined.

We could then feel sorry for people with no arms, no legs or no eyes.

We could then feel sorry for people with no home, no family, no one to lean on and assist them, even as they're facing death.

Importantly, we could learn more from those brave people. We could learn how they achieved the strength and courage to challenge those difficulties. We could learn how they stood up and thrived even from the darkest fates. We could learn from their examples, to be braver, bolder and tougher against all life's odds.

THE VALUE OF GRATITUDE

In life, we have many things to be grateful for: our breathing, foods, water, our senses, family, friends, and people who helped us in difficult times. Gratitude is to remember and appreciate what we receive from the world and other people. Gratitude is to show our appreciation for our own existence today.

Normally, we receive help from others from time to time. When we encounter a failure or disappointment in life, many times it's our family, friends, or even strangers that helped us. Even when someone pushed us down, we learned the hard lessons so that we could rise up and improve ourselves. We don't need to always blame everyone and everything around, because it's those hard times that taught us and helped us grow the most.

Deepest inside, we're not ungrateful people. However, life often creates so much stress, anxiety and hassles that we don't even notice how much we've been given in life. That's something we should learn to improve if we want make our lives happier and more meaningful.

Gratitude can be expressed everywhere, in every situation. It may simply be thinking about hard-working farmers when we eat our foods. It may simply be paying respect to our ancestors, who spent their whole lives working to bring us peace and prosperity today.

Every day, we can show our gratitude to those people who helped us in the past. We can show gratitude to our parents who gave us life. Show gratitude to our teachers who gave us knowledge and wisdom, to people who encouraged or supported us in down times. When we express our gratitude and start to help others, we could receive much more from that later on.

In our modern day, when many of us live with anxiety, exhaustion and anger, spending more time to express gratitude is of utmost importance. It's because gratitude can provide a variety of great benefits to your life:

1. Gratitude helps improve your mental health

Express your gratitude. That will help increase your happiness and alleviate depression. Gratitude is an antidote to negative emotions and difficult times in life.

2. Gratitude helps you enjoy positive experiences

We can immediately remember ten happy events in life. However, often we're too busy to spend time thinking about them. Even when good things are happening right now, we're too distracted with other matters that we often forget to take a pause and enjoy the moment.

Gratitude can help you recall great events in life, thereby generating positive feelings associated with those moments. You can make your lives happier and more positive by reliving these events and enjoying the exhilaration of those happy moments. By giving more attention to your thoughts in the present moment, you can attract more happiness as well as enjoy your senses and experiences.

3. Gratitude helps you cope with stress and adversities in life

Trauma, stress and negative events can obsess and distract our minds from positive things. By reminding ourselves of positive aspects of our situation, we can deal with our negative emotions more effectively. This will help us gain a better and greater perspective to think about a solution to the current problem.

4. Gratitude improves your confidence and self-esteem

Gratitude allows you to think about your past achievements, about the kind people who helped you along your path to those successes, as well as the blessings you received along the way. When you focus on these things, you will realize how great your life has been so far, and how much you have achieved in life. By being grateful to your skills, hobbies, and interests, you will be able to feel your inner power and improve your self-esteem. Instead of focusing on your failures and negative events, focus on many wonderful things that you can strive for and achieve in life.

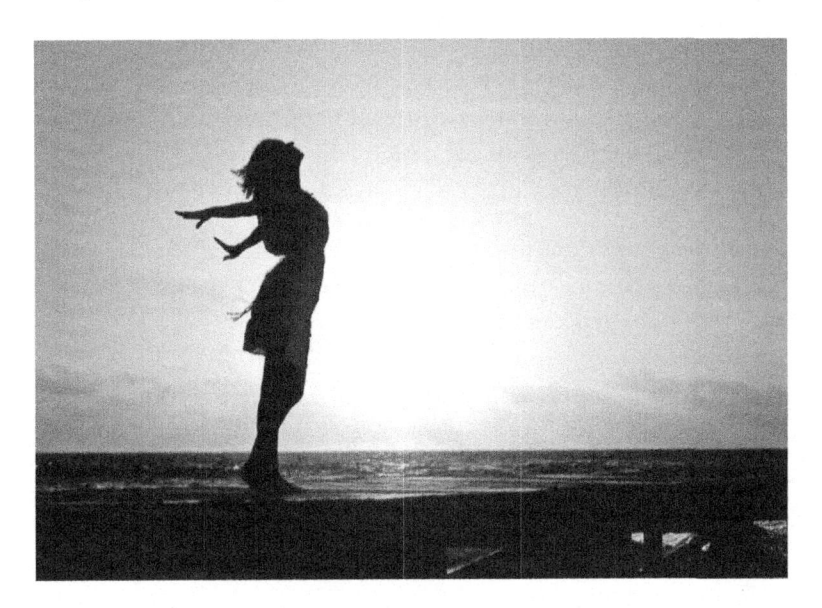

5. Gratitude nurtures compassion

When you're truly aware of what you have in hand, you will deeply understand the pains of other people who don't have it. For example, being grateful for having foods and water will allow you to be inspired and help other people. Expressing gratitude by taking concrete actions will help you be more empathetic to others' sufferings and become happier.

6. Gratitude enhances our relationships

Generally, when we want to improve our relationships with other people, we can express our gratitude to them with thanks, kindness, and support. However, sometimes just the feeling of gratitude towards someone can help enhance the intimacy and connection to that person. And as we feel connected to those important people around us, we will appreciate and enjoy our lives much more.

7. Gratitude improve mindfulness

Every time when you're carried away by stress, pains and anxiety, focus your attention on gratitude. Focus your mind on your breathing and the flow of joy inside your heart. Feel grateful for being alive. Focus on what you do have that many others don't.

Focus on your beautiful memories in life, and take a big smile. With the gratitude that many people don't even have the opportunity to experience similar experiences.

8. Gratitude is a powerful antidote for negative emotions

By being grateful for the life you have, you can now feel your peace and happiness within. By being grateful for all the good things as well as all the bad things that made you stronger, you will gradually overcome stress and worries in life.

You will then accept and appreciate everyone and everything the way they are.

You will then live in freedom with all the goodness of life in mind.

And instead of worrying so much about the future, you can now spend your precious time creating it yourself.

9. Gratitude can change your whole life's perspective

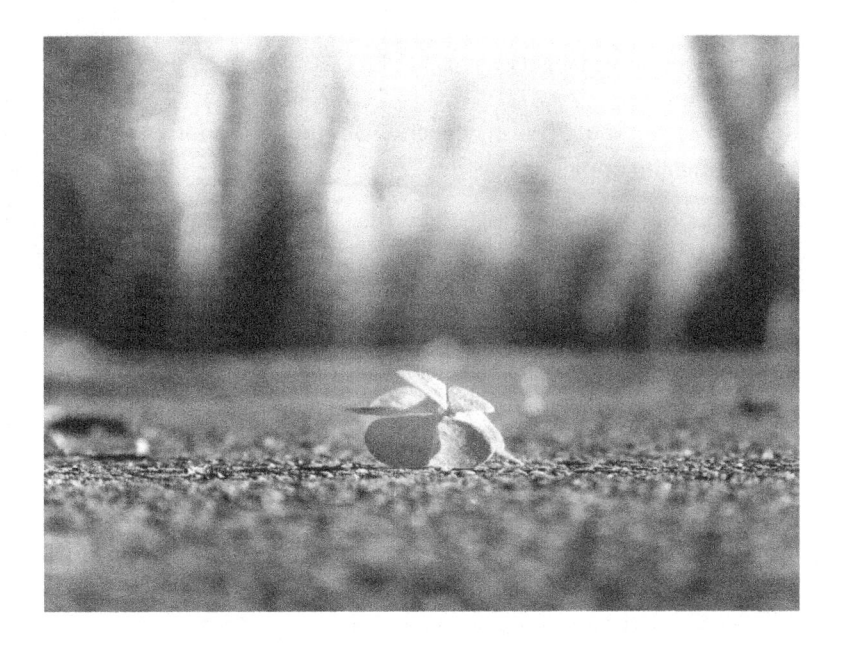

If you've ever experienced an extremely threatening situation in life, recall it.

Recall the moment you encountered or barely escaped the accident. Recall a moment of extreme fear, worry, agony, or a time of experiencing a matter of life and death. Recall those moments that you were so lucky of being alive in one piece.

At the brink of death, was your life's perspective changed? Did you begin to look at life and appreciate it more than ever?

Remember the time of having a leg injury that you couldn't walk for days? How frustrating was it?

Now you can start taking each step with extreme joy and excitement from your heart.

Remember a time of sickness, of excruciating pain and headache?

How traumatic was it?

Now you can feel glad and grateful for every second of normality. In fact, being normal isn't trivial at all.

Remember a time of stomachache, of hunger and thirst? How exhausting and appalling was it?

Now you can start enjoying every meal, every cake, every sip of wine. Like never before.

Remember a grave period of life, when everything in life seems to be against you? How stressful and difficult was it?

Now you can start celebrating each moment of comfort, of freedom and peacefulness inside.

Recall the worst times you have experienced in life, and contrast those to this present. Observe how far you've come, and how wonderful you've survived them all. Feel your gratitude for that. And let the darkest past light up your present.

Let that gratitude be the ultimate guide for a brighter life ahead.

10. Gratitude can change the way you live, and love

Gratitude can change the way you cherish each passing day.

Seeing people struggling in a wheelchair, you can feel thankful for each step you go. You can then walk, jog and run like having a new life. You will then never take a step on Earth the same way again.

Witnessing many animals being killed for foods, you can feel their agony and appreciate your better fate. You can then be thankful for each frugal meal you have. You will then never take a simple meal for granted again.

Witnessing people struggling with painful diseases, dilemmas, and even death, you can feel thankful for your current state. Since no matter how bad your life has been, there's always someone who's experiencing it more painful, more heartbreaking, and more excruciating than yours.

You will then be able to take a deep breath, and relax your soul.

You will then be able to get out of your worries, anxiety, and cherish this very moment.

Gratitude is sweet, truly sweet!

Just let yourself appreciate the wonderful world around, and feel that sweetness of gratitude burying deep inside.

Feel that extreme freedom.

Feel that sweetest love, that bliss of life, that delight of heart,

For being still luckier than many others.

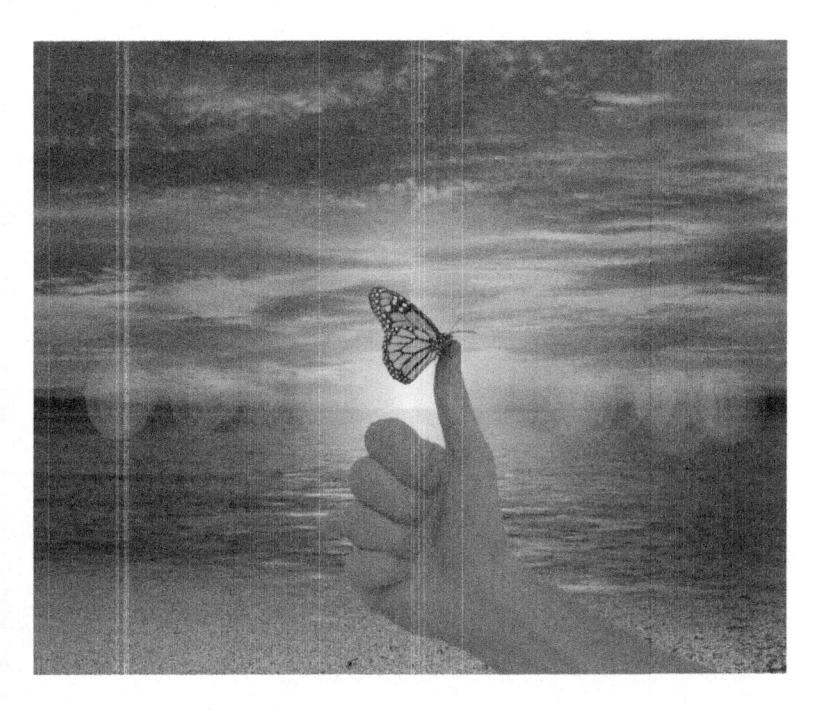

PRACTICE GRATITUDE

Gratitude is a critical ingredient of a great life. Here are some helpful ways you can practice each day to boost your gratitude and happiness:

1. Practice your "Thank You Ritual"

Say "Thank you so much, My Life" before eating, working, sleeping, and after waking up. Recall the agonizing lives of many people out there throughout the world. Recall your life's gifts that many others wish for.

Remind yourself of 5 greatest things you have that many people don't, and 3 wonderful activities that you can do today.

2. Say "Thank You" to other people

Appreciate every little thing in life that you've taken for granted. Thank those around for serving your meal, for the help and kindness that they offer. Thank them for the nice service they've given you.

3. Find inspiring examples

Find examples of people who overcame extreme hardships in life by reading books or watching the news, especially when you're feeling down or discontent with life.

See the lives of many people that are worse than yours. See how bravely they've been fighting against all life's odds.

Recognize that you're still luckier than many others.

That you can live more boldly and bravely than ever before.

4. Imagine losing something you've taken for granted

Imagine losing your friends, your legs, your arms, or your eyes.

How woeful would it be? How would you live then?

Remind yourself of all the things you have that many others don't.

Remind yourself to enjoy every step, every shape, every color and sound.

Don't wait until you lose someone to start giving love.

Don't wait until you lose something to appreciate its worth!

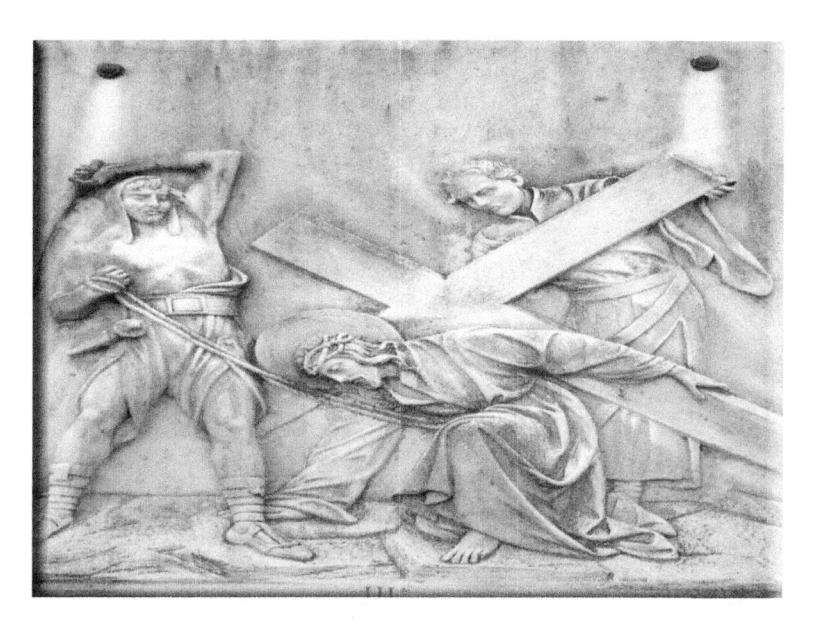

5. Take responsibility for everything in life

When bad things happen, let's refrain from blaming life and other people. Let's take responsibility for planning and taking the next step. This way, we can get more control over our negative emotions.

Then take a look at what we have, and tell ourselves: "Many people out there are living with even worse pains and sorrows, and I'm much luckier than them. So I can definitely overcome this current state. It's all my responsibility to find a better solution. It's all my responsibility to find my way back to balance!"

6. Fall in love with every little thing

Fall in love with whatever you have. Every little thing!

Adore your bed. Fall in love with it. Feel sorry for people who are sleeping on rainy streets.

Take a deep breath. Feel the peaceful joy of it. And feel sorry for people who are painfully taking each breath every passing day.

Look at your fingers. See how wonderful they are? Fall in love with them. Cherish each of them. And feel sorry for people who don't even have hands.

Today, indulge in your own senses. Savor each taste, each sound, each sight, each step you take.

Cherish the gift of being right now, right here,

And the wonder of living this life.

Be alive.

Truly alive!

6

FINDING ONE'S LIFE PURPOSE

It's not enough to have lived. We should be determined to live for something.

- **Winston S. Churchill**

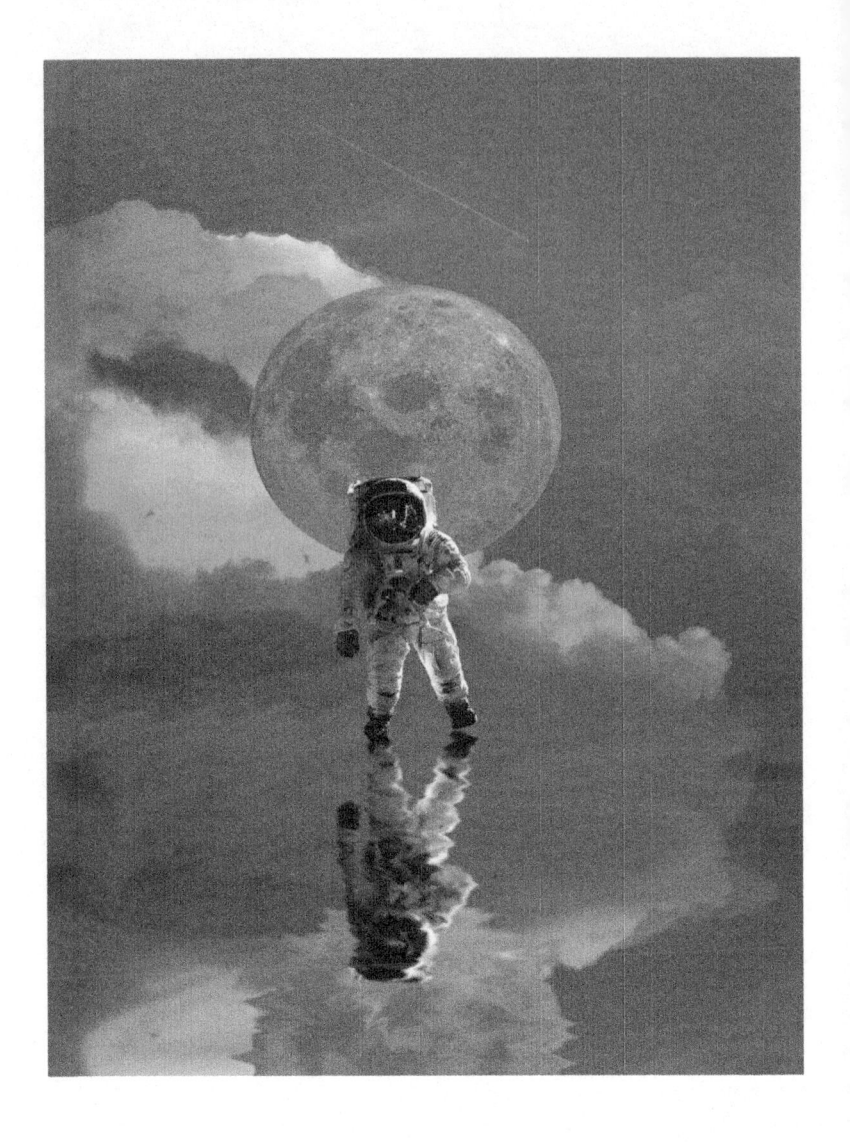

Who are we?

Where do we come from?

What's the purpose of our life?

These are the questions that people often ask themselves during free time. The truth is, no one has the ultimate answer. Nor can anyone. This is because everyone might have a different perspective on life. Everyone might have a different life purpose.

As it turns out, finding one's own purpose of existence can be very difficult. That said, it is a vital step to achieve happiness and meaningfulness in life.

Everything around us exists for a reason. Vehicles for transportation, books for storing knowledge, TVs for our entertainment, etc. For animals, every species take a specific role in the food chain, which would be severely affected if that species were lost. The question is, what purpose do we exist for in this world, apart from our dominant role in the food chain?

In the past, our ancestors' purpose was very simple: to survive and to have as many children as possible. Basically, their mission was clear: to feed and to breed. To achieve that, our ancestors strived every day to seek for foods and avoid predators. Later on, when our species dominated the world, climbed to the top of the food chain, meals and safety were no longer a big problem. Along with those great benefits, however, we lost the very reasons to exist, which had accompanied us since the beginning of our species.

In war time, life purpose was very clear. People had to choose, either to fight for their lives or die. There were very few choices available. Nevertheless, people in war time had a clear vision and goals, which were highly specific and inspiring. Against every odd and every pain in war, as such, people moved forward relentlessly each day.

After the war, however, many soldiers returned home with an

empty sense of life. In peacetime, most of them cannot find a goal that's important or motivating any more. Hence paradoxically, although people no longer have to face constant fears of death and pain, they usually feel lost with a decreased life quality.

This is very similar to the fact that after working in a project for a long time, we often feel lost when it suddenly ends. We might feel empty and have no idea of what to do next. Similarly while at work, we usually know exactly what to do, which is the tasks given by our boss every day. After retirement, however, no one gives us specific goals and missions any more. Many people hence struggle to find something to do till the end of their lives.

An existential crisis that is.

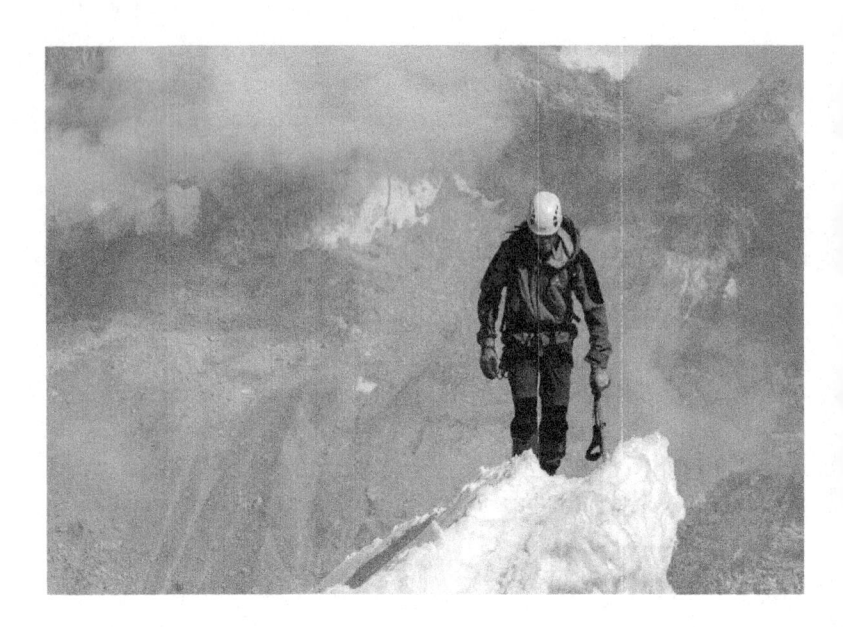

HOW TO FIND ONE'S PURPOSE

Having an inspiring purpose in life is thus a vital mission. There were many painful deaths and sacrifices during wars, but people usually lived with lofty passion and purposes, hence finding their lives highly meaningful. In the time of peace, however, every day often passes by monotonously. Common goals such as money, a high status and a romantic relationship are generally good, but they're often not inspiring enough to ignite the fire inside one's heart. And without that inner fire and passion from within, life ultimately seems empty and boring like death.

That's why nowadays many people often find it difficult to enjoy their lives. Our task, therefore, is to find the ultimate mission of our lives - the ultimate purpose, as well as several inspiring short-term goals to strive for each day. The more motivating and exciting these goals turn out to be, the more we can fully live and cherish each moment on Earth.

For example, there was a man who was struggling with the question, "What do I live for?" Years after years, he couldn't find the answer. The more he tried to find it, the more he felt lost and empty in life. Then one day, he was diagnosed with a severe illness. At that moment, he realized that he only wished to live and live healthily. He realized that his life purpose was to help others and cherish the only life he had. In the hindsight, he lost many years finding a thing that he had already possessed.

People's life becomes highly directional when they have a clear purpose in mind. March 21 is the world's Down Syndrome day. If you asked any parent of a Down-Syndrome kid, they would say their purpose in life is to take care of their children, to help them have a better life. People living in pains and adversities often find their life purpose to be helping themselves and helping others to overcome hard times.

Similarly, if you asked a mother from a poor family if she has a purpose in life, she might easily tell you. Her purposes might simply be to get her kids something to eat and go to school like many others. The mother has to make sure next week they'll have enough foods, and next month she'll be able to pay the bills. Those purposes inspire her to work hard and sacrifice herself for the needs of her children. Busy and stressful as her job may be sometimes, she can feel a great sense of meaning and happiness in life.

As it happens, often during difficult or painful periods that people find the purpose of their lives. To be a normal person having a normal life is now something they never take for granted. The lesson is that, we can learn to appreciate and enjoy what we already have. Ultimately, no matter how incomplete we have been, our life is still the life that many people wish for. Many of them would willingly swap with us if they ever had a chance!

Hence, take our time to appreciate the life we're granted. And learn to discover more purposes to strive for. If your life is empty or boring right now, find new goals, new people and new missions. Find what suits you in life. Add more spices and make it richer.

Here are the questions you can ask yourself to find out your life purposes:

If you had a free life, without any worry from money and time, what would you do?

What kinds of activity have particularly inspired you since you were a kid?

What kinds of subjects do you often pay attention to in your free time? Global warming, science, self-development, music, history?

Recall some exciting activities in the past that made you forget to eat and sleep. What are they about?

I hope you'll discover more about yourself and find your life purposes. Shape your journey into a rich, meaningful and fulfilling one. After all, we don't need to wait for life to hurt us to find out our purposes. We can always find meaningful ways to enjoy and cherish our life. Even right now.

LONG-TERM AND SHORT-TERM GOALS

In the best-selling book "Wild", Cheryl Strayed recounts the story of her own life. Feeling lost after a divorce and the death of her mother, Cheryl decided to embark on a 1200-mile journey across the Pacific Crest Trail.

It was a three-month journey of facing various dangers and difficulties along the way, but Cheryl was highly motivated. She had a clear purpose in mind, which was to finish the trail. After that, Cheryl could find her next goal: to write a book! Before embarking on the trail, Cheryl had never known about her very next step. But by moving forward relentlessly, learning new skills and experiencing new things, Cheryl could find inspiring goals one after another for her journey of life.

Similar situations happen in sports. People participating in sports often have one thing in common: they have the next goal in mind. First, to finish the race within 45 minutes, then progressively within 40 minutes, 30 minutes, etc. If there were no goals motivating and challenging enough, the activity would soon become boring and lose it meaning. The purpose of achieving a good health is not challenging or motivating enough for the activity to last long.

Similarly, when we go to work for money, money itself isn't inspiring enough. Money is merely a mean. There needs to be a deeper and inspiring purpose behind it. For instance, to take care of our family, to help others in need, or to help pursue our purpose in life. Going to work simply for money is similar to do exercises simply for a good health. No deeper purpose. No specific and challenging goals. No inner fire and passion. Boredom will definitely soon follow.

Nowadays, many of us find it increasingly difficult to do something meaningful in life. We mostly have a very similar life path, going to school, earning a degree, working, retiring, battling illness, and eventually saying goodbye. The same flow of life happens almost everywhere, in school, in office, on the street. Many of us can't even have many exciting events except the biggest milestones in life. That begs the question, "What's the point of living many years doing the same thing over and over again?"

Over the years, we've become increasingly attached to our job and family. To the point that we are reluctant to get out of our comfort zone. The need for security and familiarity is exactly what makes our life boring. I myself sometimes wish that i did use my youth more creatively and adventurously.

That said, if we cannot completely detach from our routine life, we can still make it richer. We can set exciting goals to strive for each day. Say, participating in competitive games, projects or challenges. By looking for something inspiring rather than money and status, we can make our lives far more meaningful. Because we know that we're learning, growing and conquering an inspiring challenge.

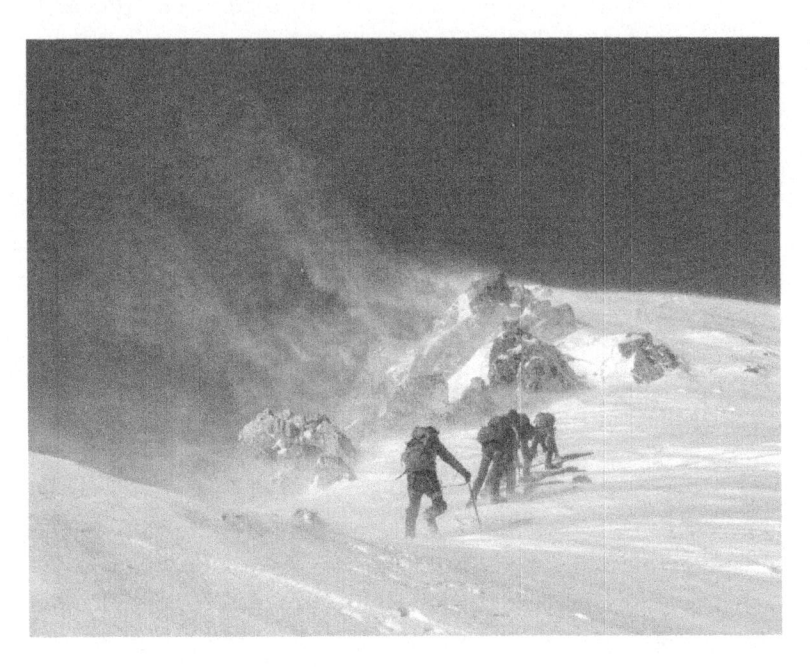

Besides, helping others is another wonderful way to live meaningfully. By helping people around us, we can feel our importance in the world. And with that, we'll feel the pride and meaning from within.

Eventually, we should have both long-term and short-term goals that excite our heart. We only need those goals to make us feel inspired and excited. We don't need them to be something big or important according to other people's standards. Why? Because everyone is different. What matters most to others may not be what excites or matters to us. What matters is that we listen to our heart and soul, to follow what can inspire us most.

Often, we say that the meaning of life is to live life meaningfully. Our meaning of life ultimately consists of our long-term vision of what inspires us in life, as well as some short-term goals that excite, challenge and help us grow. Having in mind the purpose of our life, as well as the specific actions we need to do each day is the ultimate guide to a fulfilling life.

Patty Wilson is a girl diagnosed with epileptics since a child. Her father, Jim Wilson usually practices running every morning. One day, Patty told her father that she wanted to join him, but feared that her seizures would affect the activity. Jim told her that it would be okay, since he knew what to do if such a situation happened. And so they run every day, together. The great thing happened was that Patty didn't have any seizure while running.

And then one day, Patty told Jim that she wanted to break the world record of a woman's longest distance. They checked the Guinness book, and it was 80 miles for a woman's record. At the time, Patty began her high school time and she said: "I will run from Orange County to San Francisco." It was about 400 miles. "In the second year, I will run to Portland, Oregon" (about 1500 miles). "In the third year, I will run to St. Louis" (about 2000 miles). "In the final year, I will run to the White House" (more than 3000 miles).

Patty did what she said! With the final run, 3000 miles from west to east, ended with the handshake with the US President. It was her pure determination and practice that stunned even professional athletes. She inspired millions of people and raised enough funds to open 19 centers to help epileptic patients.

In the hindsight, if Patty hadn't created an inspiring goal and hadn't taken actions to realize it, her life would have been monotonous as many other patients' lives. But simply by having a challenging and exciting goal to strive for, every day in her life turns into a meaningful one. That was a goal that requires a lot of effort and determination to accomplish. But it inspires not only Patty but every one of us. There are many other examples of overcoming pains, losses and adversities with sheer purpose and determination that are worth admiring and learning from.

THE PURPOSE OF ONE'S SUFFERING

One effective way to overcome difficult situations in life is to find a purpose for your own suffering.

For example, when you met a person who was rude to you, maybe she'd been going through a stressful period in life. She needed you. She needed your understanding and forgiveness. So maybe having to deal with her rudeness was your opportunity. It was to understand and help her. It was your purpose.

Or maybe, you're experiencing a terminal illness in life. It's no doubt very difficult to overcome the initial stress, sadness and depression. However, you can take it as an opportunity to write a book, to compose a song, to leave a legacy in the world, to help others, or to prove how strong and resilient you can be to your God. Those would be your purposes to fight for each day. Very powerful purposes indeed.

Finding a purpose or an opportunity behind every hardship will help you accept the situation and give meaning to your life.

Genuinely believe that everything happens for a reason, and that your hardship is serving a great purpose in life. That way, you'll find peace and passion in every step along your path. You'll be able to enjoy a happier and more fulfilling life.

For now, just embrace the life you have. Find out its purposes.

And make it truly rock!

7

WALKING TO ULTIMATE HAPPINESS

The purpose of life is not to be happy. It is to be useful, to be honorable, to be compassionate, to have it make some difference that you have lived and lived well.

— **Ralph Waldo Emerson**

No one is useless in this world who lightens the burdens of another.

— **Charles Dickens**

The best way to cheer yourself up is to try to cheer somebody else up.

– **Mark Twain**

Generally speaking, the most miserable people I know are those who are obsessed with themselves; the happiest people I know are those who lose themselves in the service of others. By and large, I have come to see that if we complain about life, it is because we are thinking only of ourselves.

— **Gordon B. Hinckley**

Many days, we might feel lost and lonely among billions of people. Our trouble seems so big that it often feels like there's no way out. Our headache seems so huge that it often feels like the end of the world.

During these difficult times, it would help if we could pause for a second. It would help if we could take a look at people with conditions worse than ours, people with no arms, no legs or even no eyes. As we do that, we could get a better perspective about our situation, and our problems would turn into something trivial. We could at the same time find happiness in helping people and making this world a better place. We could find our life's meaning in sympathizing with others' pains and helping them move forward.

THE SWEETNESS OF GIVING

Helping people is sweet. Not only does helping someone benefit the taker, it can also bring joy and happiness to the giver himself. When we give away or help people, our brain releases neurotransmitters that make us happy. That's why we feel sweet as we give. Giving or helping others generates one of the best emotions we can experience as a human being.

So, share your joy with others. Share your smiles and happiness to those in need. For sharing can inspire your life, and loving can sweeten your heart.

Lending a hand to someone in need will let you get out of your own personal thoughts. As a consequence, it will help you out of your agonies, negativity, and unhappiness.

Giving or helping someone will allow you to make a difference in the world. It will let you feel your worth and pride from within.

You don't have to simply exist and die. You can live great. You can live and create a lasting change.

You can make a difference. You can die with your name admired. You can die with your life remembered. You can die while living in the hearts of many people.

Today, take your chance to give away. Don't hesitate if you can offer a help. Whether it's a homeless man, a lonely child or a disabled person, you can bring smiles and happiness to their painful worlds. And with that, feel the love inside you soar high. Let the flame of loving, of existing and of being alive burns inside your heart.

Give and help. That doesn't mean that you must give everything you have. Just give what you can. Alternatively, you can raise funds, share the news, and reach out for more help.

Having a bad mood now?

Think of some ways to make a positive difference to the world. Think of some ways to **solve** problems and **serve** people.

Think outside of yourself.

Then start doing something. Create smiles and happiness for others, and you will get your smiles and happiness in return. You will get your energy, excitement, inspiration, love and all goodness in you back. You will gain more self-worth, pride and confidence that could forever change the way you see yourself and the world.

Every day, take a minute to feel.

Feel sorry for many unfortunate lives out there in the world. And feel thankful for being luckier.

Feel happy that you are able to help. Feel great that you can give away with love.

Feel delighted as you grow and deepen your caring heart.

Feel proud of your own worth.

And appreciate the value of your existence.

LOVE WHAT YOU DO

Having no motivation doing your job?

If so, don't look at your job as something you need to do just for a living.

Your job is always more than that. It's a chance for you to bring happiness to others, to bring values to this world. It's a chance for you to contribute and make it a better place.

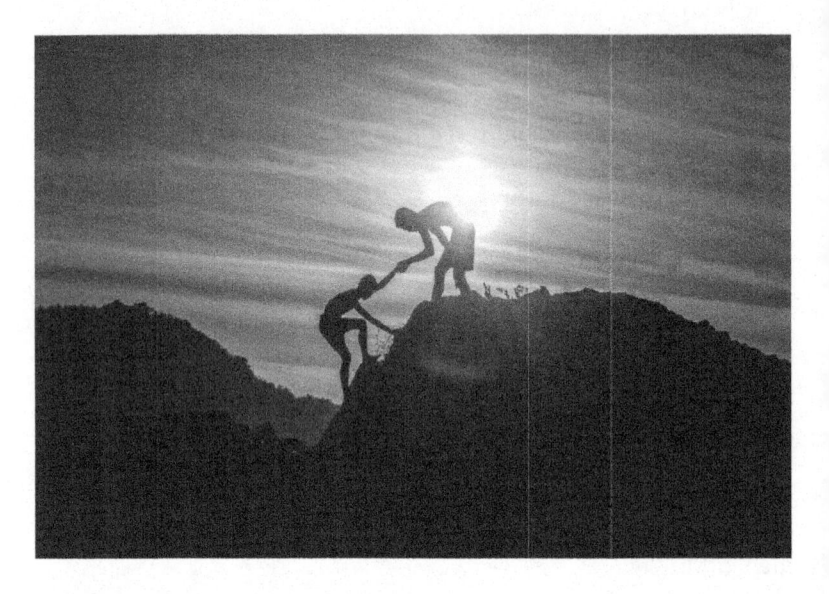

Change your own perspective. Think about what you're doing as something really important. Think about your job as something to be proud of. It's not all about money. It's not all about salary. It's about helping people. It's about changing the world. It's about proving the true value of your self.

What you do can bring happiness to other people and make this world a better place. What you do can really matter!

When you only think about what you can gain from doing your work, you can lose motivation quickly. Your brain might trick you into thinking that it would be better to sit relaxing and enjoying life now. Ultimately, thinking about what you can gain is a poor source of motivation.

Think about the values you can bring to the world instead. Think about the love and happiness you can bring to others. That way, you'll have a lasting source of motivation. You'll get a powerful push that can help you move on and overcome any obstacle or procrastination in life.

You're a seller? It's not all about selling and earning. It's about making the world a convenient and comfortable place. It's about bringing a better life to everyone. You now need to think of some ways to serve customers even more. People need you. Many lives need you. And that's great!

You're a floor cleaner? It's not all about cleaning and getting paid. It's about making the world an orderly and hygienic place. It's about serving and making others happy. You now need to think of some ways to bring more satisfaction to clients. People need you. Many families and offices need you. And that's great!

You're a teacher? It's not all about teaching and receiving salary. It's about building and shaping the next generation. It's about motivating and inspiring students for a greater good. You now need to think of some ways to motivate and help more students. People need you. Many parents and children need you. And that's great!

TAKE IT AS A PLEASURE

Every day at work, think about your job's positive aspects. See it as something invaluable. Make it a great chance for you to serve and shine brightly.

That means you don't have to wait for the tasks you're working on to be over and start enjoying life. You can now take it as an opportunity, a pleasure, and a privilege. You can now start appreciating and loving it.

Be passionate about what you're doing. Take your job as a

passion. Take it as a precious opportunity. Take it as leisure during weekend. And look forward to enjoying it even more.

Right now, find out what values you can bring to this world. Find out what great paths you can pave to honor your existence.

Stop wondering about what you can gain. Stop thinking of what you can get.

Instead, start thinking about other people's problems. Start asking how you can help.

Whatever you need to do, create for yourself a great inspiration to start.

Just ask yourself:

How can my work help people?

How can my job bring smiles and happiness to this world?

How can my sacrifice give me a great worth and pride?

Today,

Cherish what you possess.

Enjoy what you do.

Find ways to help others.

Appreciate your own worth.

And make it a life worth living!

THE ULTIMATE PATH

Happiness is elusive. We all want to achieve it. We all want to be happy in life. But often, the more we try to achieve happiness, the more evasive and out of control it becomes. The more we focus on finding happiness, the more upset and frustrated we feel about our life.

Trying to achieve happiness seems pointless. Going after it seems to be of no use.

Why is it so?

Truth is, the more we focus on finding happiness, the more we're obsessed with ourselves. And as we're obsessed with ourselves, the more personal benefits we'd like to have. When we contrast our high expectations with an imperfect reality, as a dire consequence, the more unhappy and dissatisfied we'll feel about ourselves and our lives.

That, paradoxically, is the reason why focusing on finding happiness or any personal benefits can mentally harm you in life.

If happiness is not a good choice to focus on, then, what should we look for?

What should our life's goal be?

Often, happiness may come from different sources. For example, watching TV, going for a drink, spending time on social medial or other kinds of pleasures may bring you short-term happiness. Spending time with someone you love may bring you a more stable form of contentment. Having a great life that makes you feel worthy - a life that helps this world become a little bit better – may generate meaningful and long-lasting happiness.

As such, living a life with inspiring purposes is the best way to achieve enduring happiness. It's living a life that matters to you and also to the world around. It's living a life with a cause greater than even yourself. Then, not only will you find peace and beauty in life, but love, cheerfulness and satisfaction will also suffuse your soul.

Therefore, create your path with purposes and helpfulness. Plan your way with an inspiring meaning. Make it a life that not only serves yourself, but also serves other people and a greater cause.

Then, happiness will come to you as a consequence of such an inspiring life.

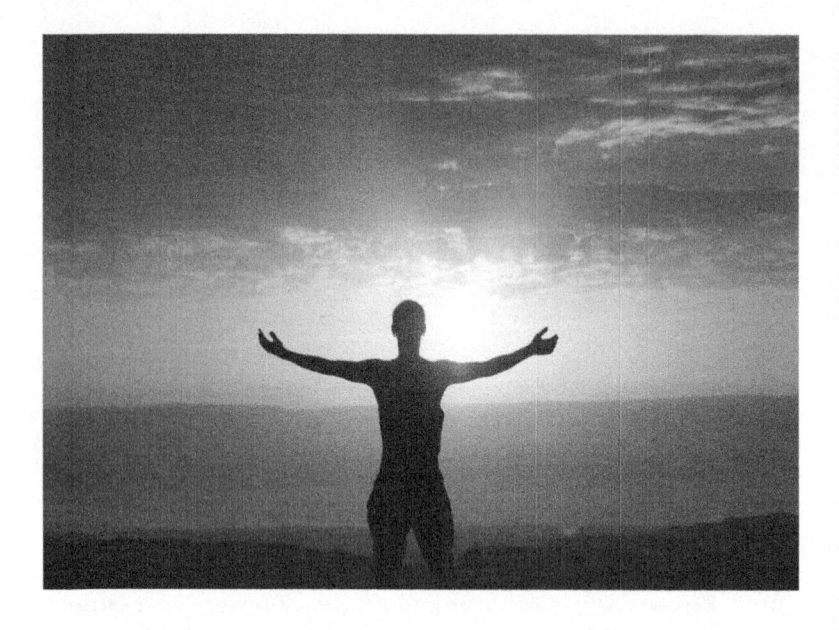

To be happy and satisfied in the long term, counterintuitively, you shouldn't think about how to achieve happiness. You shouldn't think about how much you can benefit yourself in life.

Rather, pave your way to make it a beautiful life - a life full of love, helpfulness, and purposes.

For instance, ponder upon how you can help your family, neighborhood, country, or the whole world. Think about how you can fall in love with art, science, nature, the environment, or helping other people and creatures around.

The key is to focus your attention on a cause greater than yourself. Focus on getting out of your personal boundary. Focus on helping this world and making it a little bit better.

Don't think about happiness. Don't think about how you can benefit yourself in life. Instead, think about how to offer. Think about how to serve.

Then create a proud, beautiful and inspiring goal that you can strive for and sacrifice for. See every obstacle in life as something that makes you stronger and more powerful, so that you can ultimately achieve your beautiful purpose. See every challenge in life as a necessary step for you to grow up and get to the selfless road. Afterwards, all you need to do is simply create a feasible plan and take all needed actions.

And perhaps, on the way towards that inspiring dream, you'll see happiness accompanying you. You'll feel your love. You'll feel your life's meaning. You'll feel yourself merging with other creatures, in a beautiful and purposeful walk we all call LIFE.

8

TAKING CONTROL IN THE FACE OF ADVERSITY

Accepting personal responsibility for your life frees you from outside influences, increases your self-esteem, boosts confidence in your ability to decisions, and ultimately leads to success in life.

— **Roy T. Bennett**

Much like anyone else, sometimes my life is filled with pains, losses and negativity. Sometimes it's hard to accept many things and many people the way they behave. Sometimes it's hard to move on in life with a stressful mind, with a painful past and a gray future ahead.

And my usual response to these painful times would be, naturally, to look for an outside source of the pain. It feels very tempting to blame someone or something else for whatever happened, and ignore whatever I can do afterwards.

I blame my parents as they don't give me the understanding I need.

I blame my friends for not giving me enough help and support.

I blame my spouse for not giving me the love and encouragement I want from her.

But this kind of response is extremely unhelpful. My problem remains unsolved. My mind is gradually torn apart. And it's constantly filled with sadness, anger and negativity.

Life seems to be a dead end with many uncontrollable things outside.

I feel hopeless.

For instance, when I get hurt by someone's words, I can easily blame that person for being so cruel. I instantly feel the urge from within to get angry and then complain. It's so easy just to stop there without any further action.

But if I just stop there and never take my responsibility to do necessary things, the problem will just come back. Over and over again.

So while being hurt is definitely not my fault, stopping people from hurting me in the future is still my responsibility. I need to come up with some ways to gain more respect, deal with that person's behaviors, or simply stay far away.

The difference between fault and responsibility is that fault comes from something already happened, while responsibility comes from the control of our thoughts and actions, from this very moment onwards.

Truth is, merely focusing on whose fault it was is never helpful. It simply obsesses our minds with the pains of the long gone past, and grants us absolutely no power over our future fate. Merely living in the pains of yesterday could never help us solve any problem, or bring us any closer to ultimate happiness. And while the pains of the past might happen out of control, it's still our responsibility to let go of their obsession and march bravely forward, while planning our next steps in life.

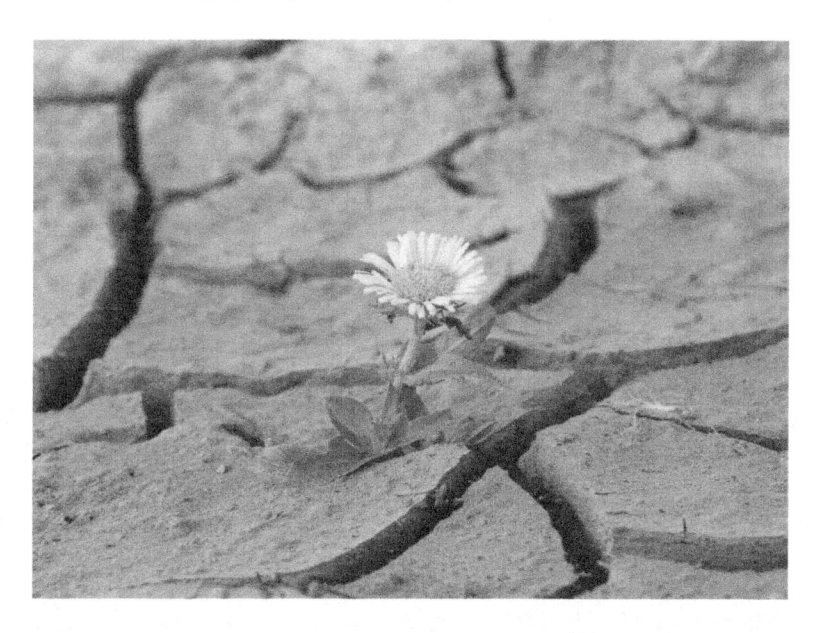

With that in mind, we can start refraining ourselves from blaming and complaining. We can take responsibility for our own thoughts, and protect ourselves from the obsession of yesterday. We can finally accept whatever happened in the past and take the wheel of our future. We can devise a detailed plan and take determined actions to reach for a happier life ahead.

Ultimately, as we realize that we can do something about a situation, no matter how small it is, we'll feel a sense of control from within. And this feeling of being in control is, indeed, the ultimate master that could help us overcome any hardship and negativity that come.

For a start, we can ask ourselves:

Is there any part have I have contributed to cause the problem in the first place?

If yes, what should I do to prevent similar problems in the future?

And what should I do if it happens again?

Given that a hurtful event already occurred, what can I do now to move forward?

What plan can I have to make my life better?

What course of action did people with similar tragedies use to survive, and even thrive?

THE POWER OF TAKING RESPONSIBILITY

Taking responsibility for everything happened is a powerful way to improve the quality of life. Here's why:

Responsibility helps you take charge of any situation

When something bad happens, we have a tendency to blame and complain about outside factors. While this might help us feel good about ourselves for a brief moment, it's devastating in the long term. It's because as we focus so much on external things, we'll feel passive and powerless against the things that we cannot change. Instead, by focusing on what we can control and what we can do, we can ultimately be more active and gain more control to improve the situation.

Responsibility helps you accept and deal with everything

When you take full responsibility for your own situation, you can learn to accept things as they are, and establish new plans to adapt to the situation.

That way, you can become adaptable and flexible. You don't need this world to be exactly how you want it to be. You can now take charge and improve your life instead.

Responsibility helps you learn valuable lessons in life

Every struggle has its own lessons that we can learn from. By focusing on learning from those lessons, we can develop better strategies and avoid similar situations in the future.

For example, if someone were rude to me, my natural tendency would be to get angry and focus on the negative aspects of that person. However, I could take my responsibility and learn something from that. I could learn to accept the person as he is, and punish his behavior by having polite yet serious conversations about the matter, or avoiding him all together if that eventually doesn't work.

In this example, you couldn't control the person's behavior when it happened.

You couldn't make him nice or respectful when he didn't want to.

But fortunately, from now on you can control how you respond to his behavior.

You can control what to focus on, either his bad behavior, or what you can learn, and what you can do to stop it from happening again.

From now on, you can control what you think about a situation. You can see it as a hopeless struggle against the world, or a great opportunity to learn your skills and renew yourself.

From now on, it's all your choice. You can choose to be either stuck with a victim mentality, or to be a passionate learner and the ultimate master of your life.

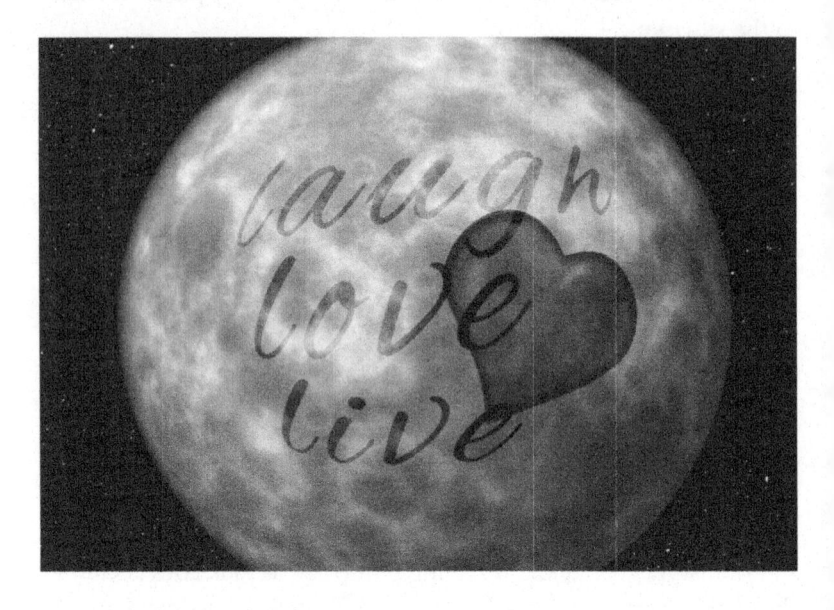

ACCEPT THE PAST, AND MOVE ON

The past is already the past. The past is already behind. And I don't need to blame anyone or anything anymore.

Why?

Because from now on, I can let go of the gone past. I can take control of my own thoughts and actions. I can start making my own decisions. I can start shaping who I am, and what my life will become.

From now on, it's MY way.

From now on, it's MY life!

9

THE ANTIDOTE OF HATE

We always expect God and others to forgive us, but many of us don't have it in their hearts to forgive others.

— **Edmond Mbiaka**

Be pitiful, for every man is fighting a hard battle.

– **Ian Maclaren**

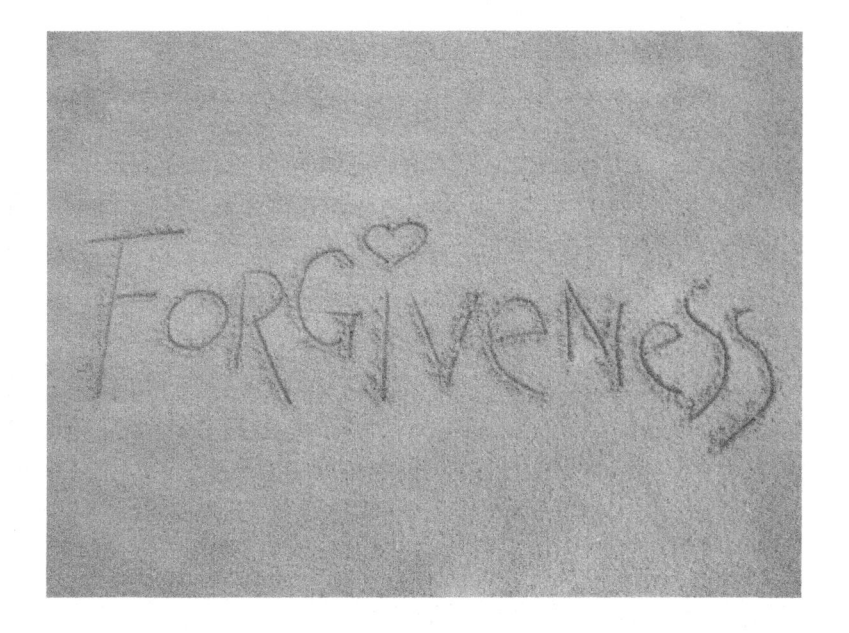

Forgiving someone can often be incredibly hard, especially if the person left a traumatic wound inside your heart. It's very difficult to forgive, not plainly because the reality of the event was inherently bad. It's difficult because the painful event left an emotional trauma inside your heart. And emotions are, after all, the ultimate masters that create the meaning of our lives and drive our behaviors most of the time. Especially negative emotions.

Especially the feeling of anger and hatred towards the person who caused us extreme pains in the past.

Forgiving someone could be very difficult. Incredibly difficult sometimes.

That said, forgiveness is always a critical ingredient for any happy and peaceful life. It's because we can't be angry and happy at the same time. We can't live happily without acceptance and forgiveness. We can't live a fulfilling life with a mind holding grudges against other people.

Anger could easily consume us. Anger could easily trap us inside if we let it to.

Eventually, we'll realize that it's so difficult to forgive, yet it's so vital have peace in life. Forgiveness, therefore, is an important skill that we need to acknowledge and constantly apply.

Now think about your life. If there's any event that keeps obsessing your soul, it's now time to ponder upon the matter, and approach it with the right mindset.

Say, if the problem is a trivial conflict, simply let it pass by "agree to disagree". Because it's liberating to accept people the way they are. It's better to accept people's dark sides as well as appreciate their good ones. Let's accept their strengths and weaknesses, as much as we can often accept ours.

Let's accept people for who they are. Because sometimes it's hard to change someone. Because we are not born to satisfy people's expectations, nor are they born to satisfy ours.

However, if you find yourself unable to accept someone's behaviors, you can find some ways to make them more aware of what they've done. You can try talking to the person, addressing your concerns, helping them understand, and hopefully, behave better. You can always learn the right methods and strategies to deal with different types of behaviors, thank to books, counseling, and other valuable sources of help.

And lastly, if you feel you can never accept someone, and cannot find any way to make that person behave better, just relax. Forgive him. Then simply walk away and move on with your life.

Forgive. Always forgive. That will help you keep the peace inside your heart.

"Why should I forgive such a horrible thing?" You might ask.

Because of PEACE. Because you and your beloved self deserve it!

Because forgiving someone doesn't necessarily mean that you must always keep them in your life. You can always choose some appropriate actions. You can always accept people, try to change them, or just simply walk away.

You can always have a choice.

Forgive. Then focus on loving yourself and your beloved ones. Focus on giving love to other people in need. Focus on your hobbies, dreams, and life purposes instead.

From now on, you can love and take care of yourself. In knowing that you deserve peace. You deserve to be free from darkness. You deserve to be free of ill will and hatred. You deserve to have a great and peaceful life.

In order to be free, you will need to believe in yourself. You will need to believe in your own strength and courage to defeat the ego's tendency of hatred and revenge. You will need to believe in your own power to love and forgive others.

You will need to choose happiness and tranquility, in spite of the painful yet long gone past.

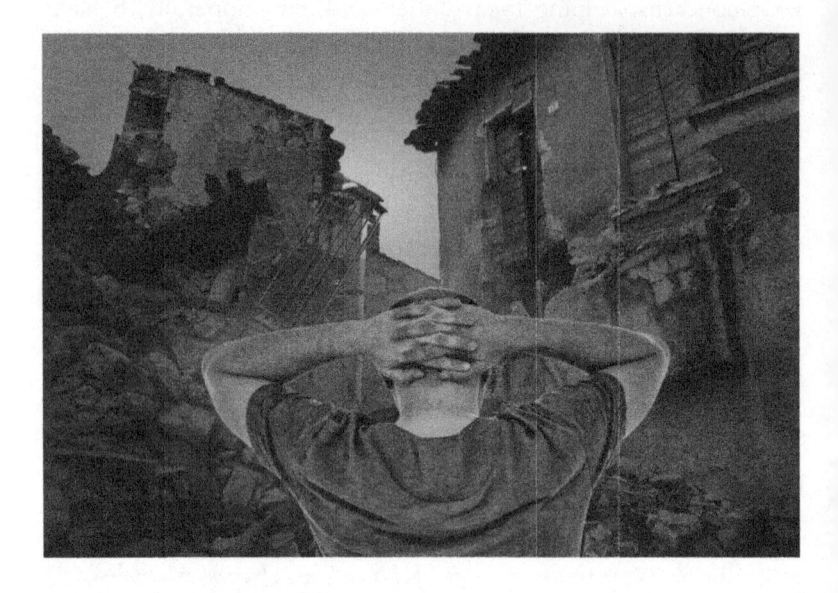

And remember that people's negative behaviors are often their problems, not yours.

Maybe they're sick or feeling down.

Maybe they're just having a bad day.

Maybe they were mistreated and had agonizing pains.

Maybe they were poorly raised and spoiled by other people.

Maybe their genes affect and predispose them to be that way.

Maybe they're wrestling in extreme stress with their own lives.

Therefore, their rude behavior towards you might be a signal of distress. It was a call for others' help. It was a call to someone who could give them a hand and pull them out of darkness. And the person they chose to ask for help was you.

After all, you can always choose to pierce through any external event, to see the real inside world, to understand the emotional needs and causes of any behavior. You can always refuse to look at people and things just from the outside.

And it would help if you could pause a second, and ask them: "Am I causing you troubles, or you're just having a bad day?"

Every time people do bad things, they might regret and suffer later. Every time they make a mistake, it's their own sin.

It's their problem. It's their guilt.

Not yours!

So, don't take things too seriously and too personally. Maybe it's not about you. It's about them after all.

Moreover, remind yourself that we all make mistakes in life. Recall those times you did things wrong in the past. Recall those times you intentionally or unintentionally hurt others in life. Recall how much you regretted afterwards. Recall how much gratitude you had as you were forgiven.

With that in mind, you can now forgive others in return. Because **who knows, if you were in their shoes, maybe you would make it even worse**. If you had experienced what they'd gone through, maybe you would've behaved even worse!

So, don't ask yourself how people could behave that way. Ask yourself what life situations, feelings and experiences could explain their behaviors. Ask yourself how you can help them out. Give people the chance to regret, to learn, and get better.

Forgive all. And move on in life with love.

Be yourself. Don't let others' rudeness make you rude. Don't let people change how kind and awesome a person you can be. Don't let them change the way you love and cherish your own path.

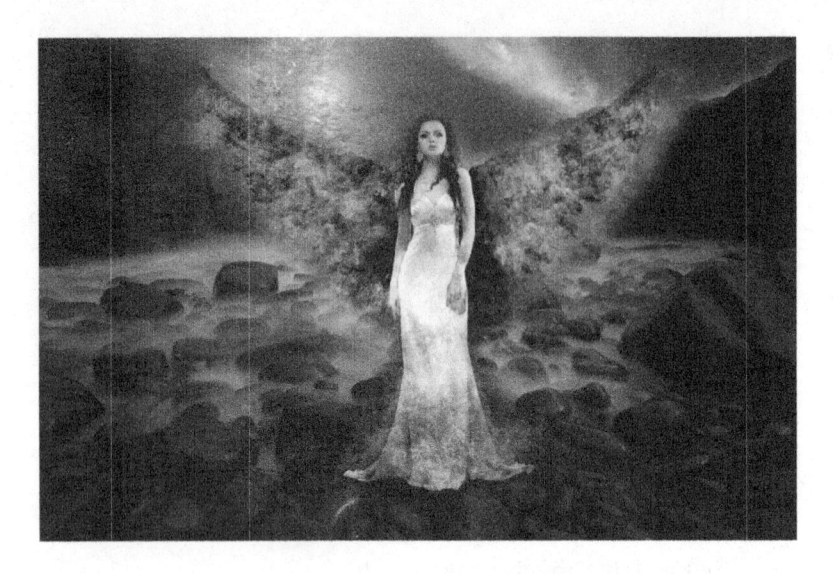

Right now, imagine you and those people you hate were all going to die. Approaching death, they all would regret so much, and would say sorry for their wrongdoings. So take your chance to forgive and be benevolent. Take your chance to live and be your best self.

Take your chance to live the few days you have left in love. And pure love only.

After all, the past is something already happened. The past is pretty much over. As such, it's your joy and your happiness now that really matter.

It's your life and your love now that really matter.

Imagine those who mistreated as angels. They're all in fact angels disguised in the form of bad guys. The universe has sent them here to offer you a unique chance to grow. They've been here to make you wiser and stronger. They've been here to test out your true love.

Thank you so much, angels!

10

OVERCOMING LAZINESS AND PROCRASTINATION

Procrastination is one of the most common and deadliest of diseases and its toll on success and happiness is heavy.

- Wayne Gretzky

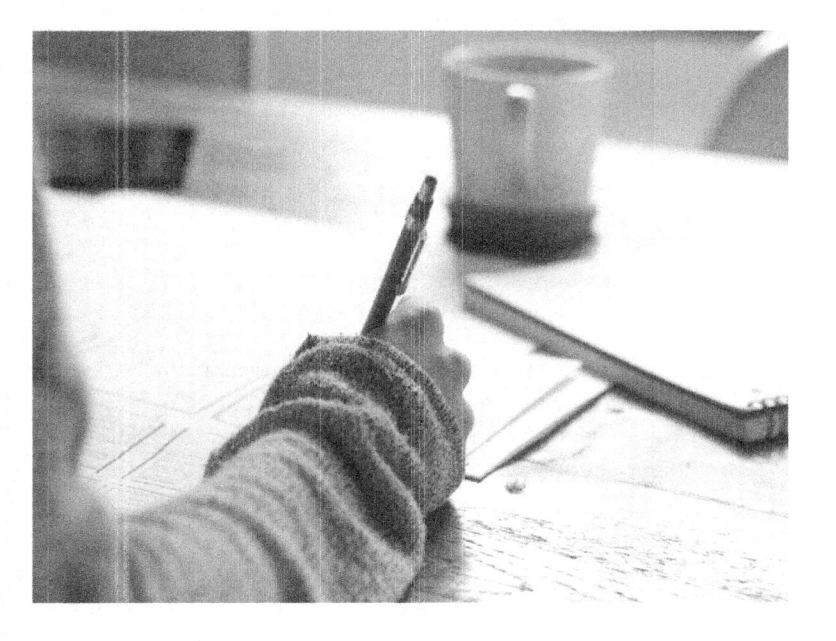

Short-term pleasures, such as having a snack, watching TV or surfing social media, are often one's favorite modes of activity. In fact, human brain is wired to look for activities that bring about short-term pleasures. Usually, they bring us temporary satisfaction and happiness. We therefore have no difficulty convincing ourselves to find some reasons and excuses, allowing ourselves to indulge in the fun of those activities.

We often overestimate the importance of those short-term pleasures, and ignore other tasks that are more significant in life.

On the other hand, long-term success comes from achieving our dreams and aspirations. It is a process which is both challenging and rewarding. Achieving our long-term goals gives us better self-esteem and life satisfaction. Getting to our long-term dreams gives us a great sense of pride and happiness.

As often, however, obtaining our long-term goals turns out to be very tough and difficult along the way. We have to acquire a huge amount of knowledge and then think of a feasible plan. We have to start taking actions and spend a massive amount of effort on finishing tasks. We have to overcome all kinds of distractions, procrastination, stress, discomfort, and fears.

To be successful in life, therefore, we'll need to confront and go through all worries and pains. We'll need to overcome every doubt and uncertainty. We'll need to live with discomfort and bitterness so that one day we can enjoy the sweetness of glory.

Hence it's crucial to focus on our long-term goals each day, and frequently remind ourselves of what we really need to do. We need to focus our mind on the thoughts of what we aspire and how we can get it. We need to think about the reasons why we must achieve those goals, how they are connected to our deepest life purposes, and how they can serve ourselves and others.

We need to remind ourselves to start taking action. Right now. No matter how small an action it is. We need to have a plan for every day. Then just focus on each day, each moment, and totally ignore the remaining amount of tasks we have to conquer in the future. We need to consider taking action right now a great success itself, and simply do it.

And no matter what difficulty lies ahead, we know we can learn to make it through.

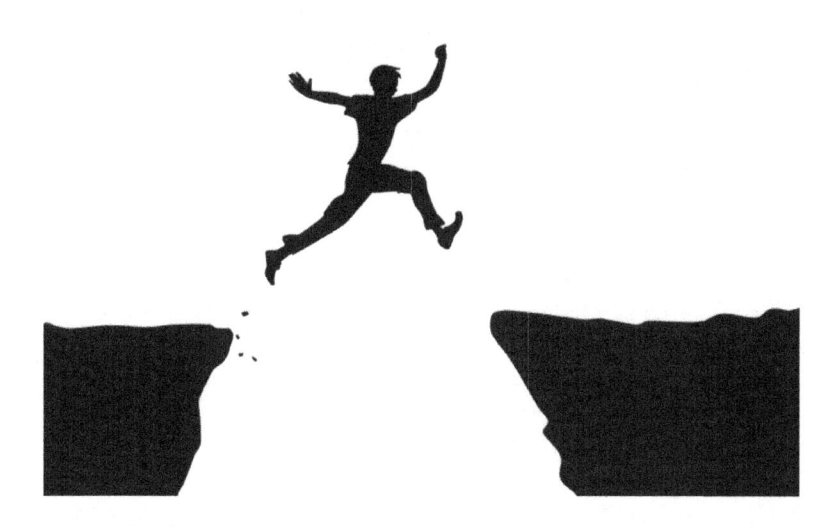

It is a natural fact that our human brain is wired to look for short-term benefits and pleasures. We're wired to avoid discomfort and pains. This tendency is, unfortunately, the main reason why it's so difficult to achieve success in life. We often find it tempting to be distracted by various sources of short-term pleasures. We easily fall into the habit of delaying and making excuses for our inaction.

Excuses are often the biggest reasons for our laziness and procrastination. Deepest inside, we know that we should not stand still. We know that we should take action immediately and regularly to achieve our goals. Yet, as always, our lazy mind bribes us to relax and have fun first. It distracts us with TV, social media and many other unimportant things.

This doesn't mean that we should ignore the joy of daily fun and pleasures.

Truth is, it's necessary to take a break each day to chill out and savor our life. We can arrange regular free time for our hobbies, to have fun and enjoy pleasures. That way, we'll be able to enjoy and appreciate every little thing we have. That includes our foods, water, each step, each sound and each sight we're able to experience.

Most of the time, nevertheless, it's crucial to concentrate on taking the action we've scheduled for each day. And even more specifically, on the action we've scheduled for this very moment.

That is the only way to realize our dream.

Indeed, we need to remind ourselves of the reasons and the purposes of our goals each day. We need to visualize the excitement, pride and satisfaction once we achieve them.

After that, let's embark on our own life' journey. Focus on taking a single and simple action needed to be done right away. Not some action in the future, but at this exact moment. Focus every thought and every effort on the present. Ignore the past and the future. If you still found yourself thinking about the past or worrying about the future, you'd need to focus on your breathing and senses to bring you back to the present.

Remember, start just by taking a little step. The simplest of all. That way, you wouldn't have to rely on your mood. You wouldn't have to wait for any motivation to come.

Because they would rarely come without first taking action.

Eventually, the act of starting, no matter how little the first step is, would help create passion and motivation to push you forward.

Right now, let's get started! Move on. And move on no matter what.

Right now, you can choose to be lazy. You can choose to procrastinate as much as you can. You can choose to go for all kinds of short-term pleasures. You can choose to look for all kinds of long-term toxins. Going this way, eventually, you would never get to your dreams. At the end of this road, eventually, you would feel guilty and hate yourself so much.

You would regret.

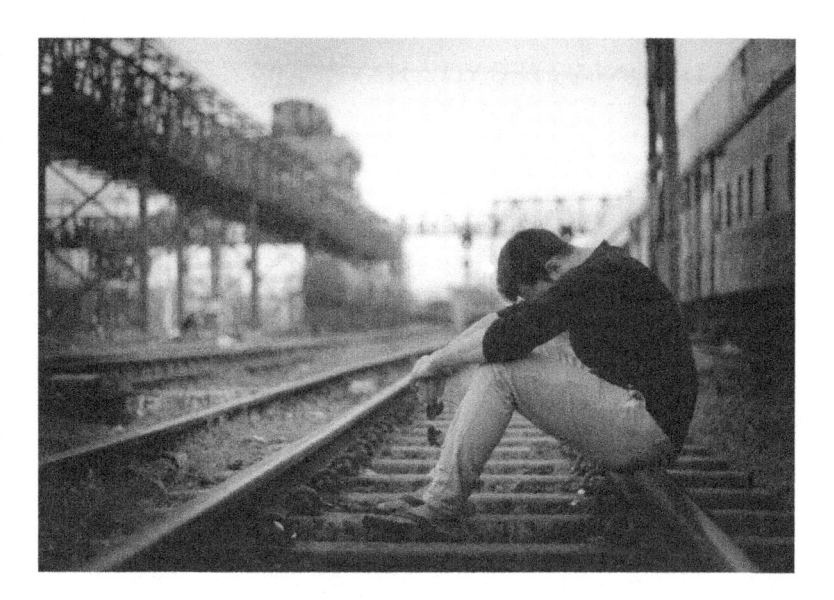

Or, **you can choose** to get up and start working now. You can choose to confront all challenges and discomfort. You can choose to endure all bitterness that many people hate. So that one day, you can savor the sweetness of pride and glory that many people lack.

For now, what you need is just the courage to get up.

What you need is just the courage to move on.

Just start.

Just ignore all temptations.

Forget all distractions.

And live with a burning fire in mind.

Live.

Truly live!

FOR THE ONLY LIFE YOU HAVE.

11

THE ONLY PATH TO SUCCESS

Inaction breeds doubt and fear. Action breeds confidence and courage. If you want to conquer fear, do not sit home and think about it. Go out and get busy.

- Dale Carnegie

In order to succeed in life, taking action is the only way forward. It's the only way to achieve one's dreams.

Here's the specific steps you'll need to take.

I. IDENTIFY YOUR TARGETS

First, think about what you really want in life.

Think about your ambitions and dreams. What do you want most? What kind of life do you want to have? What gives you the purpose and meaning of living your life?

Next, pinpoint your short-term and your long-term targets. What kinds of achievement do you want to get today? This week? This month? This year? And the next 10 years?

It's important to establish your goals as precisely and feasibly as possible. If they were too easy, you'd procrastinate and have no motivation to start. Too difficult, you'd be intimidated and surrender even before starting.

Balance is crucial.

Be specific and realistic.

Because the more you know about yourself, your life, and the road you wish to follow, the more you can take charge of your own path.

Identify your targets. Then take necessary actions to realize them. This is the path you have to take to get what you want in life.

Now, spend several minutes to ponder upon your life. Think about the kind of person you wish to be in the future. Think about the kind of life you want to have each day.

And be determined to reach for your dream. There's no point

sitting and waiting for it to come. Because most of the time, it won't! Pave your way and start taking a step towards your beautiful dream instead.

Create your future. Don't sleep until catastrophes take your down. Improve yourself and better your life actively instead. By doing so, you can stop troubles and negativity from controlling your path. Or at least, if burdensome problems already happened, you can now work your way to overcome them all. In a courageous, heroic, and proud manner.

Because the most important thing in life is that you already did your best.

II. CREATE YOUR PLAN

To achieve your dream, it's crucial to have necessary skills and knowledge.

You can begin by reading and learning from successful people. You can learn a lot from many successful stories around the world.

How did successful people achieve their goals?

What strategies did they have?

What were their daily habits?

What motivated them to overcome every failure and reach for success in life?

After having necessary mindset and skills, it's important to create a plan for the road ahead, as specific as possible.

Write down your plan, with detailed steps and clear-cut deadlines for every day, every week and month. It's important to divide a big task into extremely small parts to work on. Without "dividing to conquer", you'd soon get intimidated by the huge amount of work. You'd likely procrastinate and eventually give up.

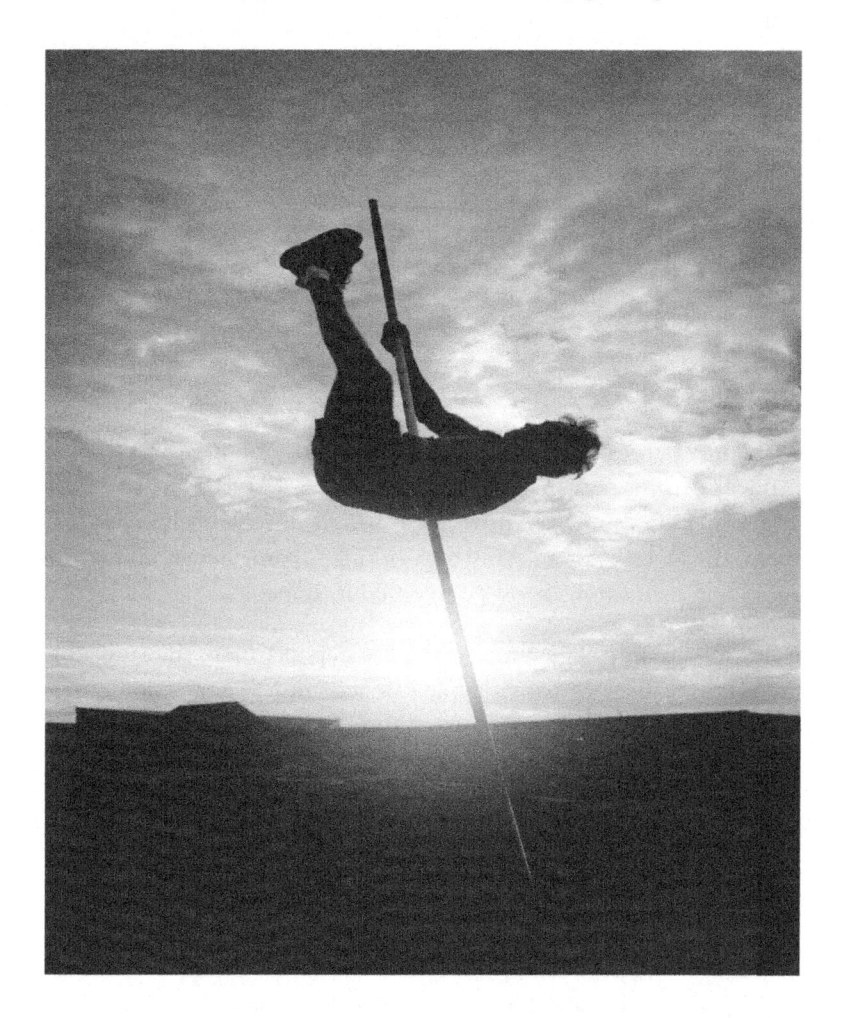

III. START TAKING ACTION

1. Believe In Yourself

To have enough strength and motivation to start, first you need to believe that you CAN make it. You need to believe in your potential, your worth, and yourself. It's important to constantly remind yourself that "If many people could make it, absolutely can I!"

On the other hand, if you kept doubting your worth, you'd soon view yourself as someone incapable of achieving the goal. If you kept hesitating to take action, your brain would soon come up with all kinds of excuses to procrastinate. You'd see the task as something impossible to overcome, and you'd eventually surrender.

To move forward, you'd need to believe in your own worth and capability. Truly believe that you can do your best and achieve great things in life.

Right now, if you are still struggling and doubting yourself, you can learn from many people who succeeded despite their bad luck and brutal fates. Learn how their beliefs in themselves helped them through the darkest walks of life, against even the most agonizing pains and sorrows one could imagine.

Believing in yourself is always a crucial step. As such, start utilizing the mindset that "If many people can accomplish it, absolutely can I!" Learning to adopt such an attitude is perhaps the most vital key to reach for one's dreams.

2. Imagine

In order to have great motivation and start taking action, it's important to imagine the feeling of getting to your dream. How glad and wonderful would you feel? Picture that beautiful moment with colors and pride. Live in the great happiness, joyfulness and exhilaration of your fabulous dream.

Cheer and honor your success. Picture yourself full of confidence and satisfaction.

Imagine your achievement. Feel it. Relish it with extreme excitement.

3. Beat Procrastination

Along your path, you'll have to deal with a lot of distractions and procrastination. They'll become huge mental obstacles preventing you from achieving your goals.

Your mind will frequently convince you to relax and do something else. It will often persuade you to take a break, reply messages or watch television, and that you don't have to rush to get your work done after all.

Your mind will give you all kinds of excuses to procrastinate. It will bribe you with all sorts of fleeting pleasures, and will take you away from your wonderful life path.

Importantly, you may not be aware of the situation until it's too late.

You'll need to help yourself out of this situation.

Remind yourself of the reasons why you started.

And tell yourself:

"Do I want to waste my life for these fleeting pleasures?

Do I want to lose the wonderful life I always wish?

Definitely not!

Instead, I am ready to overcome all obstacles, excuses and procrastination.

I am ready to make my life beautiful.

I am ready to make myself proud of my courage, strength and determination."

Take care of what you think about. Focus on what you have to do today. Focus on your dreams and aspiration. Focus on your power and control from within.

Just begin. Just step towards your future. And ignore all excuses.

Just start right away!

By simply opening your laptop, reading the first few sentences of a book, or setting the alarm clock to remind yourself, you would soon get the inspiration to do more. Always keep in mind that it's important to make the first step as easy as possible. Otherwise, you would struggle with a lot of distractions and procrastination.

4. Enjoy The Progress

To focus effectively, you would need to cut off all possible sources of distractions. Turn off the internet if possible. Put your phone away. And sit at a quite place where you can focus on your own work.

When you begin, again, remember to make it an easy start. Split up your task into tiny and feasible parts. If you feel that the current part is still difficult to do, split it up further. It's also important to concentrate on doing one part at one moment, without stressing yourself thinking about other parts. By doing so, you'd not be overburdened by the huge workload that you have to complete.

Also, challenge yourself a little by setting a working speed faster than normal. Set a deadline sooner than what you can normally finish. Make it an interesting game. Make it fun! By doing this, you would have a lot of excitement and improve your performance. You'd be able to merge yourself into the process and enjoy every little achievement along the way.

Furthermore, use great rewards to excite and motivate your mind. It could be a short walk, a few minutes checking social media, reading an interesting book or watching a favorite video. It could be anything that highly excites your heart.

It's now time to immerse yourself in the process and enjoy the game you've created. Savor the excitement of creating a proper challenge and conquering it. Then take the time to celebrate after finishing each part and reward yourself decently, being proud that you've done a great job today.

IV. CREATE USEFUL HABITS

Ultimately, the most stable and useful strategy is to work regularly and automatically. It's important to make your work an automatic habit, so that you wouldn't have to struggle to make a start every time you want.

To begin, you need to do your task regularly, ideally every day at first. Also, use the same environmental cue to start your habit each day. That could be after breakfast, when you come home after work, or when you finish doing exercises. After a few times, you'd feel the urge of doing the task automatically when the environmental cue comes up. By doing so, you'd save a lot of time and willpower fighting against your laziness and procrastination.

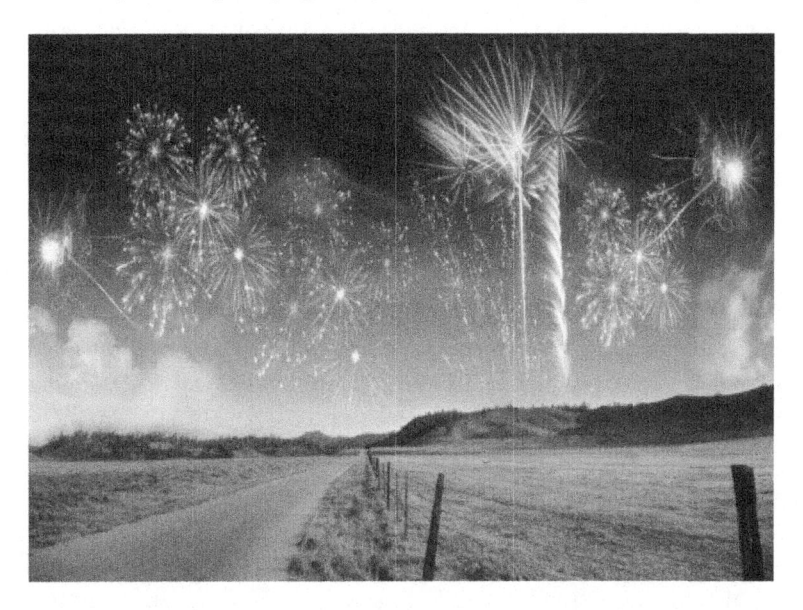

ACTION IS THE WAY FORWARD

When I was a child, I had a dream. I wished to write and publish a book of my own. However, I found it extremely difficult to make such a dream come true.

At first, I was struggling with writing so much. A long-term plan was therefore needed. Initially, I began to read a lot of books and blog posts. After that, I created a blog on my own. I could then learn to write and edit my blog posts gradually.

Eventually, when my writing was improved, I began to write the first few pages of my own book. It was still difficult at first, but I kept visualizing success in mind and getting inspired by my future accomplishment. I celebrated and enjoyed the life I wished before I could even achieve it.

Still, sometimes it seemed to be overwhelmingly difficult for me to complete the task. Many times, the thought of incapability and surrendering came up in mind. It seemed impossible for me to write a book. Procrastination, distractions and excuses all persuaded me to quit. Sometimes I couldn't write a single word during many days, many weeks and months. Moving forward seemed like a heavy burden. Finishing the work seemed like an impossibility.

Until one day, I became aware of my own limiting beliefs and thoughts. To stride forward, I was determined to adjust my attitude and believe in myself once again. I started to believe that I was completely competent and could absolutely achieve success. Furthermore, I planned to create a regular habit of writing instead of relying on my irregular mood and motivation. So for the first week, I pushed myself to sit down and write just a few sentences at the same time of each day. The same environmental cue (the moment I finished having breakfast) was used as a signal to open my laptop and start working. I also turned off the internet and removed all other distractions. Afterwards, I split the task into highly easy and small parts, and gave myself an exciting reward after finishing each session.

Gradually, I could sit down and write easily after having breakfast. It soon became an automatic action, without having to force myself to start anymore. I soon began to enjoy the mental game of challenging my limit tremendously.

I created a useful habit.

The point is, with appropriate methods and a proper mindset, you can realize your dreams too.

In fact, we always have a choice. We can choose to procrastinate and make excuses for our laziness. We can choose to be defeated by our own limiting beliefs. We can choose to believe there's truly no path to a better future.

Or we can choose the opposite. We can choose to rise up from the ashes and fight like a warrior. We can choose to rebuild our lives and future. We can choose to walk towards our beautiful dreams every day, by having the right attitude, beliefs, and actions.

Eventually, this is our life. This is our choice and our responsibility. This is the life we can better and make it more beautiful.

Every day, we need to take care of our energy and attention. Without proper eating, sleeping and exercising, we wouldn't have enough energy to stride forward. Without proper focus and attention, we'd let our minds distracted and wander far from our initial plan.

Taking the right actions is the only path we can achieve success in the future.

It's ultimately not about having ideas and plans. It's ultimately about taking the right actions every day. It's about finding a way to enjoy and indulge ourselves in the progress of walking forward.

So, readjust your attention. Don't let procrastination and short-term pleasures take you out of your path. Don't let that beautiful dream go far and you yourself regret later.

Let the excitement and enthusiasm of what you can create motivate your heart. Let the exhilaration and eagerness of what you can do inspire your day.

Wake up. Jump high. And ignite your passion.

Be patient. Be diligent. Be resolute.

And be the best version of yourself.

YOU WILL MAKE IT!

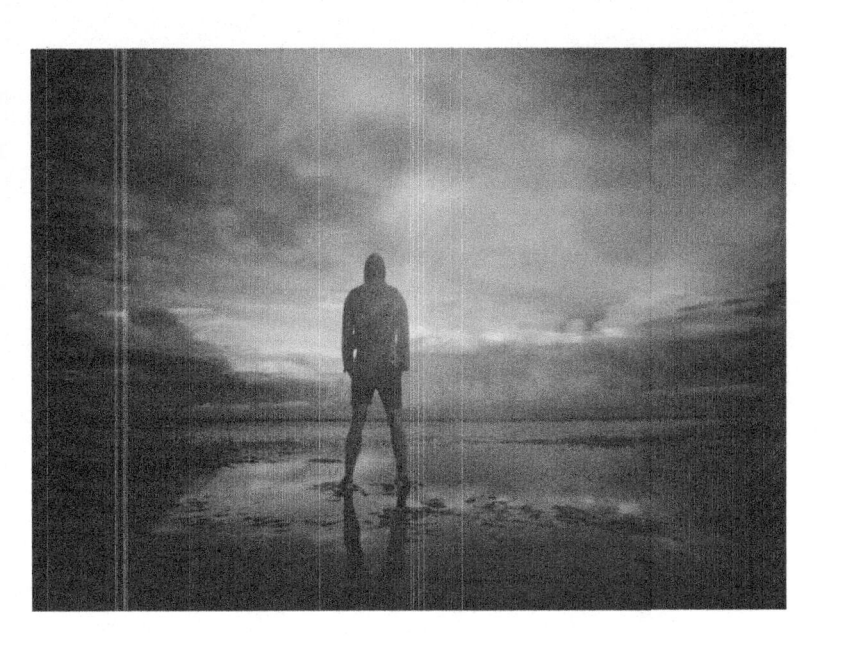

FINAL WORDS

Dear readers, thank you so much for taking a look at this book. And I sincerely hope it would give you a push in life.

I wish you all the best.

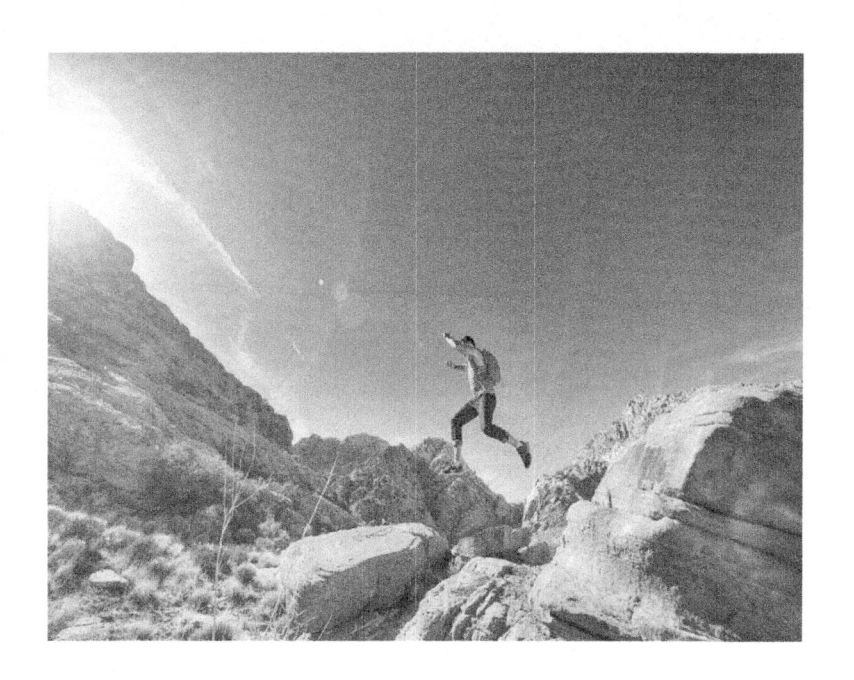

REFERENCES

The Subtle Art of Not Giving A Fuck

by Mark Manson

The Power of Now

by Eckhart Tolle

Awaken The Giant Within

by Anthony Robbins

MY CONTACT

Dear readers, please contact me via my email address (kimkhanhthan@gmail.com) if there's any inspiring story you would like to share.

Thank you so much!

RECOMMENDED READING

The Beloved
by Osho

Love, Freedom, and Aloness
by Osho

The Subtle Art of Not Giving A Fuck
by Mark Manson

Meditations
by Marcus Aurelius

A Guide to the Good Life: The Ancient Art of Stoic Joy
by William Braxton Irvine

A New Earth: Awakening to Your Life's Purpose
by Eckhart Tolle

The Tantra Experience
by Osho

Meditation: The first and the last freedom
by Osho

How to Think Like a Roman Emperor: The Stoic Philosophy of Marcus Aurelius

by Donald Robertson

Life, Love, Laughter

by Osho

Made in the USA
Coppell, TX
12 April 2021